ASTHMA

Questions
you
have
. . . Answers
you
need

Other Books From The People's Medical Society

Take This Book to the Hospital With You
How to Evaluate and Select a Nursing Home
Medicine on Trial
Medicare Made Easy
Your Medical Rights
Getting the Most for Your Medical Dollar
Take This Book to the Gynecologist With You
Take This Book to the Obstetrician With You
Blood Pressure: Questions You Have . . . Answers You Need
Your Heart: Questions You Have . . . Answers You Need
The Consumer's Guide to Medical Lingo
150 Ways to Be a Savvy Medical Consumer
Take This Book to the Pediatrician With You
100 Ways to Live to 100
Dial 800 for Health
Your Complete Medical Record
Arthritis: Questions You Have . . . Answers You Need
Diabetes: Questions You Have . . . Answers You Need
Prostate: Questions You Have . . . Answers You Need
Vitamins and Minerals: Questions You Have . . . Answers You Need
Good Operations—Bad Operations
The Complete Book of Relaxation Techniques
Test Yourself for Maximum Health
Misdiagnosis: Woman As a Disease
Yoga Made Easy
Hearing Loss: Questions You Have . . . Answers You Need

ASTHMA

Questions you have ...Answers you need

By Paula Brisco

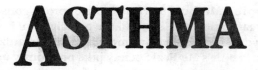

People's Medical Society.

Allentown, Pennsylvania

The **People's Medical Society** is a nonprofit consumer health organization dedicated to the principles of better, more responsive and less expensive medical care. Organized in 1983, the People's Medical Society puts previously unavailable medical information into the hands of consumers so that they can make informed decisions about their own health care. Membership in the People's Medical Society is $20 a year and includes a subscription to the *People's Medical Society Newsletter*. For information, write to the People's Medical Society, 462 Walnut Street, Allentown, PA 18102, or call 610-770-1670.

This and other People's Medical Society publications are available for quantity purchase at discount. Contact the People's Medical Society for details.

© 1994 by the People's Medical Society
Printed in the United States of America

Library of Congress Cataloging-in-Publication Data
Brisco, Paula.
    Asthma : questions you have, answers you need /
by Paula Brisco.
        p. cm.
    Includes bibliographical references and index.
    ISBN 1-882606-16-7
        1. Asthma—Miscellanea.   I. Title.
RC591.B74   1994
616.2'38—dc20   94-23176
                                                         CIP

1 2 3 4 5 6 7 8 9 0
First printing, September 1994

CONTENTS

INTRODUCTION

More than 15 million Americans suffer from asthma, making it one of the most common diseases. Its effects range from relatively mild to life-threatening cases. Each year at least 500,000 people are hospitalized because of asthma.

Asthma is not an adults-only disease. Some 7 percent of all children develop it. Among children, twice the number of boys contract asthma than do girls. Yet among adults, the disease strikes males and females equally.

What is especially startling—and worrisome—about asthma is that it is on the increase. Its reported incidence rate has increased by 60 percent in the last decade. And the number of deaths in the United States from asthma have doubled since 1978. Experts suggest that 90 percent of those deaths are preventable.

There are two important points to remember about asthma. First, as the above statistics so graphically note, asthma is a very dangerous disease. Second, asthma is treatable. And the more you know about the disease itself and the treatment options available, the more likely you are to survive and flourish.

Ironically, medical research suggests that one reason for the dramatic increase in asthma incidence and deaths due to asthma may be the failure of many physicians to properly diagnose or treat the disease. Thus, while physicians are essential partners in the treatment of asthma, complete reliance on and blind faith in them may be detrimental to your health.

In *Asthma: Questions You Have . . . Answers You Need,* we present the information a consumer suffering from asthma or their family needs to know to be an equal partner and informed decision-maker in their own care and treatment.

Asthma is a complex condition. There are several types of asthma and a wide variety of treatment options. For the average consumer, all the issues can become a confusing hodgepodge of medical gobbledygook. In this book, all the information a consumer needs to know is presented in an easy-to-use format and in understandable language.

As the nation's largest consumer health advocacy organization, the People's Medical Society is dedicated to getting helpful and healthful information to the consumer. It is our philosophy that an informed consumer is an empowered one—a person capable of making the best health-care decisions in partnership with her health-care provider.

Charles B. Inlander
President
People's Medical Society

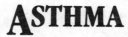

ASTHMA

**Questions
you
have
. . . Answers
you
need**

Terms printed in boldface can be found in the glossary, beginning on page 167. Only the first mention of the word in the text will be boldfaced.

We have tried to use male and female pronouns in an egalitarian manner throughout the book. Any imbalance in usage has been in the interest of readability.

1 BEHIND THE SCENES OF ASTHMA

Q: What is **asthma?**

A: Asthma is a disease in which air passages in the lungs periodically become narrowed, obstructed or even blocked. Medical science classifies asthma as a respiratory disease, because it interferes with the process by which oxygen is delivered to the body's cells—and, as you know, oxygen is necessary to sustain life.

Q: What is an asthma attack?

A: This is the term used to describe a period of breathing difficulty. People who are in the midst of an asthma attack often experience wheezing, coughing, chest tightness and shortness of breath.

Q: How serious can these attacks be?

A: An asthma attack may be so mild that the person with asthma barely notices it, or an attack can be life-threatening and require hospital care. Sometimes an asthma attack is an isolated event; other times, it is part of a pattern of daily, weekly or monthly attacks. Often, attacks become more severe as they increase in frequency, but this is not always the case. Asthma affects every individual differently.

Q: How many people have asthma?

A: Today over 15 million Americans of all ages have asthma, according to statistics released in 1993 by the National Institute of Allergy and Infectious Diseases.

Q: Do children experience asthma more than adults?

A: Most asthma develops in childhood, sometimes even appearing in infancy. Somewhere in the neighborhood of 7 percent of the children in the United States develop asthma; about 5 percent of adults develop the disease.

Many youngsters eventually outgrow their asthma; others experience an asthma-free period during their teens or early 20s but later develop asthma again in adulthood.

Adults with no previous history of asthma can also develop the disease any time from their late 20s onward. We'll talk more about childhood and adult asthma later in this chapter.

Q: Are males more likely to have asthma?

A: In children, boys develop the disorder twice as often as girls. Among the adult population, however, men and women are equally affected.

But all people with asthma have one thing in common: They have difficulty breathing.

Q: What causes breathing difficulty?

A: In general, it's caused when the airways narrow in reaction to certain stimuli, usually something inhaled. These stimuli are commonly called **triggers**. Although everyone's air passages have the potential to constrict in varying degrees, an asthma sufferer's passages are supersensitive and respond to irritants that do not affect other people. Medical professionals use the word **hyperresponsiveness** when they refer to the process of airway narrowing.

Q: What exactly causes airway narrowing?

A: To explain how asthma affects breathing function, let's look at the respiratory system of a healthy person. When someone inhales, air enters the nose or mouth and flows through the throat (known as the **pharynx**), through the voice box (**larynx**) and into the windpipe (**trachea**). The trachea branches into two tubes called **bronchi** (one serving the right lung, the other the left), which then divide into smaller bronchi, which in turn branch out into **bronchioles**. At the tips of the bronchioles are tiny air sacs called **alveoli**, which contain minute blood vessels called **capillaries**. This network of bronchi, bronchioles and alveoli is known as the **bronchial tree**.

The job of the bronchi and bronchioles is to funnel air to the alveoli, which remove carbon dioxide from the capillaries and replace it with oxygen. This is known as **oxygen exchange**, and it is the basic process by which oxygen gets into our blood. Of course, this oxygen-rich blood then travels to our hearts and through our bodies.

Q: How is the process different when a person has asthma?

A: In someone with asthma, the process of inhalation and oxygen exchange occurs just as it does in someone without the disease. However, three abnormal reactions take place when the person with asthma meets up with a trigger. These reactions cause asthma symptoms.

Q: What's the first reaction?

A: One occurs when the muscles that encircle the bronchial air passages squeeze the passages, thus reducing the flow of air. The contractions—known as **bronchospasms** or **bronchial spasms**—are tiny muscle spasms that start quite suddenly and last a relatively short period of time.

Q: What is the second reaction in an asthma attack?

A: The cells along the bronchial airway walls (called the **mucosa**, or **mucous membranes**) produce a large amount of thick, gummy mucus. Mucus is normally produced to lubricate the airways so air flows smoothly, but during an asthma episode, the amount of mucus increases substantially. The mucus collects along the bronchial walls, thus narrowing the airways. In more severe asthma attacks, the mucus may form sticky plugs that clog the air passages.

Q: And the third reaction?

A: The linings of the bronchial tubes—the mucosa— become inflamed, which makes the airways puffy and swollen. The swelling narrows the airways, restricting the amount of air that can pass through. Unlike bronchospasms, which occur over a relatively short time span and then go away, airway inflammation tends to linger for hours, days or longer.

Q: **Does every asthmatic person experience all three reactions?**

A: Yes. Some people with mild asthma think that bronchospasms and a slight amount of mucus production are their only signs of asthma. However, recent scientific research has found that inflammation is present in most asthma, even mild cases.

In short, an asthma attack is a period of breathing difficulty exhibiting three factors—bronchospasms, mucus production and inflammation. And these three combine to reduce the amount of space through which air can flow to the lungs. This airway narrowing (sometimes called **bronchoconstriction**) may worsen gradually and persist even when asthma medications are taken, but it can also develop abruptly and produce severe respiratory distress.

Q: **That's because airway narrowing makes it difficult to inhale, right?**

A: Actually, it makes it difficult to *exhale*.

Q: **Why is that?**

A: Asthma is a problem of getting air *out* of the lungs, not getting air in. When an asthmatic person inhales, the lungs pull air in and down the airways, past areas of inflammation and mucus buildup, all the way to the alveoli. However, when it comes time to exhale—normally a smooth and easy deflation of the lungs—air gets trapped behind areas of inflammation or behind clumps of mucus. These airway blockages are sometimes described as one-way "valves" that trap air in part of the lungs. When the valves are closed, it takes more effort to exhale, and the person may **wheeze** or cough with the effort of trying to force air through blocked air passages.

Q: How long does an asthma attack last?

A: Asthma attacks may last several minutes or go on for hours or even days. As an attack progresses, wheezing and excessive mucus production increase. Some attacks resolve themselves spontaneously; others must be halted with medications. The longer an attack persists, the more dangerous it is.

Q: Why is that?

A: When airway obstructions let air in but limit the amount of air that goes out, the lungs become over-inflated with stale, carbon-dioxide-laden air. Decreasing amounts of fresh, oxygenated air reach the obstructed areas of the lungs, which means less oxygen gets into the blood to nourish cells.

Q: Is this dangerous?

A: It can be. If the situation persists, carbon dioxide builds up in the body and the person may experience **respiratory failure**—meaning, in effect, he could pass out and die.

Q: How long before this severe response occurs?

A: It generally takes days or weeks for inflammation and obstructions to reach a point where oxygen transfer is severely impaired. Once that point is reached, however, breathing function can deteriorate in a matter of hours.

Q: So asthma is a disease that should be taken seriously?

A: Absolutely. It's essential to recognize the disease's signs and symptoms and act on them.

Q: Again, those symptoms are . . . ?

A: These are the most common and distinctive:

• *Shortness of breath*, an early sign of asthma, appears as a sensation of breathlessness or choking, as labored breathing or as panting or gasping for air. Known as **dyspnea** in medical lingo, shortness of breath is thought to be caused by bronchospasms.

• *Chest tightness* is a feeling of pressure in the front of the chest, in the area around the **sternum**, or breastbone. Again, this is a result of bronchospasms.

• *Wheezing* is the result of air being forced through narrowed or constricted airways. It may be loud enough to be heard by bystanders or audible only through a doctor's stethoscope. Best described as a whistling or rasping sound, wheezing is initially heard on exhalation. But as asthma worsens there is wheezing during inhalation as well.

Q: I've been told that wheezing disappears when an asthma attack is severe. Is that true?

A: You've raised an important point. The absence or disappearance of wheezing is not necessarily a sign that asthma is improving: In very severe attacks the wheezing and other breath sounds may become more and more faint as the asthma sufferer becomes extremely fatigued. If this state does not improve or is not resolved in some way, the chest becomes ominously quiet—what doctors refer to as the *silent chest*—and the situation may lead to respiratory failure.

Q: Back to asthma symptoms, please.
Are there others we should know about?

A: Absolutely. They include these:

• *Excess mucus* is produced during an asthma attack, and this thick, sticky matter obstructs or clogs the airways. Excess mucus is a symptom of asthma, but it is also a *cause* of the next symptom.

• *Coughing* occurs as the body tries to clear obstructions from the lungs. The cough may be a deep and loose cough that brings up mucus. The person with asthma may cough up **mucus plugs**, small chunks or spirals of mucus that have taken the form of the bronchioles. Or the cough may be dry and hacking. A cough that fails to bring up mucus, called *nonproductive* in medical lingo, may eventually irritate the lungs and in itself produce bronchospasm.

• *Anxiety* or *apprehension* often accompanies an asthma attack, an understandable reaction to breathlessness. The anxiety, apprehension or feeling of panic may dissolve into a feeling of exhaustion once the attack has passed.

Q: Does someone with asthma experience
all those symptoms?

A: No. Symptoms vary from person to person, and not every symptom must be present during an asthma attack.

Q: If someone has those symptoms, does it
mean he has asthma?

A: Not necessarily. Several conditions have symptoms that can mimic asthma, including **chronic bronchitis** (an inflammation in the lungs that leads to the daily coughing-up of large amounts of mucus), **emphysema** (a respiratory disorder in which the alveoli become permanently damaged),

heart failure and lung cancer. Wheezing and coughing in children may be a sign of **cystic fibrosis** (a hereditary lung and pancreatic disease). Coughing may even indicate something as simple as an upper respiratory infection.

Q: How, then, can doctors be sure someone has asthma?

A: The big difference between other diseases and asthma is that asthma attacks are episodic, whereas the breathing difficulty associated with the so-called similar conditions is mostly permanent. Thus, in diagnosing asthma, doctors look for evidence of **reversibility**—that is, indications that episodes of breathing difficulty come and go. Does the person have a hard time breathing one week but no problem the next? Do the lungs seem to operate perfectly well between attacks? Do attacks resolve themselves spontaneously or with medication? Yes answers are signposts for asthma.

Q: You're saying that a person can have this disease but feel perfectly fine?

A: Many times, yes. With asthma, if the lungs are not in what doctors call a "symptomatic state"—meaning no bronchospasms, mucus production or inflammation is causing asthma symptoms—then the person can breathe freely, and the lungs and air passages appear completely normal. During symptom-free periods, even a physical examination by a doctor may not uncover signs of asthma.

All of this is good news: It means that most people with asthma can live full and normal lives. With conscientious self-care and sound medical treatment, most people can control their asthma, reducing the number of asthma attacks and sometimes even eliminating them.

Q: It seems we hear more about asthma today than years ago. Is asthma a new disease?

A: Not at all. Asthma as a disease has been written about since the time of the ancient Greeks. The word *asthma* derives from the Greek verb "to pant," which describes the way some people appear to breathe when their asthma is active.

Q: I've read that more people are developing asthma. Is that true?

A: Sadly, yes. Despite the fact that asthma is a reversible and controllable disease, the incidence of asthma is increasing. The number of asthma patients in America has grown by more than 60 percent in the last decade, with minorities hardest hit. Deaths from the disease have more than doubled to some 4,000 since 1978. About 500,000 people are hospitalized annually because of their disease.

Although asthma, as a disease, has a low death rate compared with many other chronic diseases, its economic costs are enormous—an estimated $6.4 billion in the United States in 1990 alone. Of that, $1.6 billion was spent on inpatient hospital services and another $1 billion on medication. Despite all that money poured into medical care, adults lost nearly 3 million workdays and children missed more than 10 million school days due to asthma.

Q: Is this a problem only in the United States?

A: Actually, the same problem is being reported elsewhere in the world. The incidence of asthma in Western countries has doubled in the past 20 years. Developing nations are also seeing increases in reports of asthma.

Q: Why is asthma on the upswing?

A: Many explanations have been offered. Some experts believe that the higher numbers reflect better awareness, diagnosis and reporting of the disease. Other scientists point to increased air pollution; to the greater number of chemicals in the home, work and outdoor environment; and to factors related to city living in particular. Urban areas seem hardest hit, and the reasons for this may relate to issues of poverty: greater exposure to substances that trigger asthma and lack of access to timely and prevention-oriented medical care.

Once people develop asthma, they may not get adequate care from physicians, and some experts believe this key factor accounts for part of the increase in mortality. A reluctance to use **anti-inflammatory drugs** to treat underlying inflammation, the misunderstanding of the role of allergies as triggers, a lack of physician training—these contribute to the inadequate treatment of the disease, says Michael Kaliner, M.D., chief of the allergy section of the National Institute of Allergy and Infectious Diseases. "In terms of hospital care, medicine and lost work and school days, asthma is a serious and expensive disease that could be treated more cost-effectively with preventive measures and improved care from primary physicians," he says.

Another asthma culprit may be related to the foods we eat—or, more precisely, don't eat.

Q: How is that?

A: New research suggests that changes in diet in Western countries may be leading to a greater incidence of asthma. According to a 1994 report in the *British Medical Journal*, children today are eating less fresh fruit and fish. These foods are important sources of vitamins C and E and coenzyme Q, nutrients thought to have a role in proper airway function. Their deficiency in the diet could lead to more airway blockage and inflammation.

Q: Is asthma contagious? Could that be a reason it is more prevalent?

A: Absolutely not. You cannot "catch" asthma from someone.

Q: Is asthma psychosomatic?

A: No. The myth that asthma is "all in the head" was once widespread in the medical profession. Even today some physicians remain convinced that a person's asthma is more of a psychological problem than a physical one—an attitude some doctors assume when the treatment plan they recommend proves ineffective.

It's important to realize that emotions and stress do play a role in making asthma worse, as we will see in Chapter 2, but they do not produce asthma in someone who doesn't already have the disease.

Q: Is asthma inherited?

A: People do not inherit asthma per se, but they may be born with a genetic predisposition to develop the disease. *May* is the operative word here. The chances of having the predisposition to asthma are greater if someone in the immediate family has asthma—a parent, sibling or grandparent.

Q: What are the chances of inheriting the predisposition?

A: One 1993 study found that in families with one parent who was hyperresponsive, close to 28 percent of the children had the same condition.

Obviously, the more blood relatives with asthma, the greater the chance a child may be born with a predisposition to asthma. In addition, people with a family history of hay fever or allergies stand a greater chance of having the asthmatic predisposition. But having a family history of asthma, hay fever or allergies does not guarantee that a person will develop the disease.

Q: **Is there any research on the role of genetics in asthma?**

A: In 1992 two British scientists said they had identified a gene that causes asthma. However, five other studies could not confirm the existence of such a gene. Work continues in this arena, because researchers believe that, if true, such a finding could lead to improved asthma treatments within a decade.

What studies have confirmed is that people inherit a susceptibility to develop asthma, which may then be galvanized by factors in the home, work or outdoor environment.

Q: **Is there a test to determine whether someone will develop asthma?**

A: Not yet. Medical science has yet to devise a way to spot asthma before it appears in its classic manifestation: shortness of breath, chest tightness, wheezing and coughing. Even if there's a strong family history of asthma, doctors can't tell whether it will develop, if it will be intermittent or chronic, when it will become active or what will trigger it.

In children, however, a skin problem known as **atopic dermatitis** is often a red flag for asthma in the future.

Q: What is atopic dermatitis?

A: This is a long-lasting and sometimes severe form of eczema, an itchy red rash that can appear on the face, wrists, elbows, backs of the knees and ankles. One in ten children develops atopic dermatitis. According to Hugh Sampson, M.D., writing in *Understanding Asthma: A Blueprint for Breathing* (American College of Allergy and Immunology, 1990), about half of those youngsters with atopic dermatitis later develop asthma; about three-quarters of the children develop asthma, hay fever or both. Like asthma, atopic dermatitis is provoked or exacerbated by triggers that may include allergies, dry skin, skin infections, sweating and stress.

Q: You mentioned earlier that there are different types of asthma. What are they?

A: Over the years, the medical profession has developed several ways of classifying asthma and of distinguishing one form of the disease from another. Let's take a look at some of these classifications now.

Traditionally, doctors have separated asthma into two general categories, **extrinsic asthma** and **intrinsic asthma**, depending upon the types of stimuli that trigger episodes of the disease.

EXTRINSIC ASTHMA

Q: What is meant by extrinsic asthma?

A: Asthma triggered by allergies is known as extrinsic asthma. It is also called **allergic** or **atopic asthma**. In this form of the disease, an asthma attack is clearly linked to the body's response to something inhaled or, occasionally, ingested. Substances to which the person is allergic are called **allergens**.

Q: What sorts of things can be allergens?

A: The most common allergens are tree and grass pollen, **mold**, animal **dander** (pieces of sloughed-off skin, much like dandruff) and **dust mites**. We'll talk in detail about allergens and other triggers in Chapter 2.

Q: Who develops extrinsic asthma?

A: Asthma that develops in childhood is likely to be extrinsic asthma. Over 90 percent of asthmatic children under age 16 have allergies, as do 70 percent of asthmatic people ages 16 to 30, says Michael Kaliner of the National Institute of Allergy and Infectious Diseases. Symptoms of extrinsic asthma often vary seasonally and occur intermittently. In more than half the cases of extrinsic asthma, there is usually a personal or family history of other allergies, such as hay fever and skin conditions.

INTRINSIC ASTHMA

Q: What is this?

A: Asthma that develops in people over the age of 30 is usually intrinsic or **nonallergic asthma**. As the names imply, this asthma is not allergy related.

Q: What, then, is it related to?

A: Triggers such as respiratory infections, exercise, stress, inhalation of chemical irritants (such as cleaning fluids or fresh paint) and air pollution. While doctors believe that extrinsic asthma is caused by an overactive immune system, they don't yet understand the origins of intrinsic asthma.

Q: Is it important to know which form of asthma I have?

A: Insofar as it helps you understand your disease and suggests a path for medical treatment, yes. However, you should be aware that most people with asthma have both forms. For example, it's very common for someone with the extrinsic form of the disease to experience asthma attacks when she has a cold or the flu—both intrinsic triggers.

Extrinsic and intrinsic are two terms that attempt to describe the source and trigger of the asthma. Other types of asthma have been named after the particular situations in which they occur, such as **nocturnal asthma**, **seasonal asthma** and **exercise-induced asthma**.

NOCTURNAL ASTHMA

Q: What is this?

A: Nocturnal asthma is the name for asthma that suddenly worsens in the middle of the night, often between 2 and 4 a.m.

Q: Is this common?

A: Very. Although an asthmatic episode can happen anytime, day or night, researchers who chart trends have discovered that attacks occur more frequently at night and early in the morning. Results from surveys in England and Scotland suggest that about 50 percent of asthmatic people are awakened in the night by an asthma attack at least 20 times a year, 70 percent wake at least one night a week, and some 85 percent have occasional sleep interruptions.

Q: Who gets nocturnal asthma?

A: Nighttime asthma affects people with extrinsic and/or intrinsic forms of the disease.

Q: What causes it?

A: Scientists have not yet uncovered the "mechanism" behind nocturnal asthma, but they have several theories. One theory points to obstructions caused by mucus in the airway walls of someone with asthma. This mucus is less likely to drain or be cleared naturally when that person is lying down. Instead, it accumulates in the bronchial tubes, obstructing airflow.

A second theory blames exposure to allergens in the bedroom (such as dust or animal dander). But this does not explain the problem in people with nonallergic asthma. A related hypothesis says that nighttime symptoms may be the result of a delayed reaction to exposure to an allergen hours earlier in the day.

Q: Are there any other theories?

A: Yes. A third theory links nocturnal asthma to **circadian rhythm**, the body's natural 24-hour cycle, which causes nighttime fluctuations in hormone levels. Blood levels of epinephrine and cortisol, two hormones that help keep bronchial tubes open, fall between midnight and six o'clock in the morning. **Histamine**, a natural chemical that worsens asthma, reaches its highest levels during the night. These factors, plus other changes related to circadian rhythm, may act as triggers for nocturnal asthma attacks.

Whatever the cause, nocturnal asthma should be taken seriously by the asthmatic person and his physician, particularly in light of surveys showing a high frequency of respiratory arrest and death due to asthma in the early morning hours. While these problems certainly don't happen to everyone who experiences nocturnal asthma, at the very least, loss of sleep can affect performance at school and work and make asthma more of a burden.

SEASONAL ASTHMA

Q: Is this a form of asthma that happens only at certain times of year?

A: Yes, although the particular season varies from person to person. Seasonal asthma is linked to extrinsic, or allergic, asthma. Some experts think that it strikes most frequently in the summer, which would explain why asthma deaths are almost 15 percent higher in summer than during the rest of the year.

EXERCISE-INDUCED ASTHMA

Q: This is asthma caused by exercise?

A: Yes. Anyone who has ever had shortness of breath, chest pain or tightness, wheezing, coughing or endurance problems during exercise may have experienced exercise-induced asthma. Estimates of asthmatic people who have had a bout of exercise-induced asthma range from 65 to 100 percent.

Q: What causes it?

A: Exercise-induced asthma is caused mainly by bronchospasms. Experts think they result from the loss of heat or water or both from the lung during exercise because of the rapid inhalation of air that is cooler and drier than that of the airways. Bronchospasms can come on as quickly as a few minutes after exercise starts. Exercise-induced asthma generally reaches its peak 5 to 10 minutes after stopping the vigorous activity, and usually disappears 20 to 30 minutes later. Because untreated exercise-induced asthma is disruptive, medications are often prescribed to prevent this type of attack. We'll talk about these medications in Chapter 4.

Q: Are there other types of asthma?

A: Medical professionals are now adopting a more descriptive classification system, built around the frequency and severity of symptoms. The two main categories are **intermittent asthma** and **chronic asthma**.

INTERMITTENT ASTHMA

Q: What is this?

A: While asthma by definition is episodic, meaning flare-ups come and go, people with intermittent asthma (also called *occasional asthma*) have extended symptom-free periods. Their symptoms may last five days a month or less, then they may go months without experiencing any sign of asthma. In between attacks, such people lead normal lives.

Seasonal asthma sometimes falls into this category of intermittent asthma.

CHRONIC ASTHMA

Q: Does this refer to more frequent asthma attacks?

A: To be precise, people with chronic asthma have symptoms for long stretches at a time: more than five days a month for more than three months and more than half of the days in any one month. People with chronic asthma go for long periods in which they have trouble breathing. Their lungs don't completely recuperate between attacks.

Q: All this is confusing—I just want to know how to tell if my asthma is severe. Is there help?

A: Yes. To help health-care practitioners diagnose asthma and devise sound treatment plans for medical consumers, the National Asthma Education Program developed detailed asthma-management guidelines in 1991. Devised specifically to educate primary-care physicians, its report divides chronic asthma into three subcategories according to severity. In adults, the three are defined as follows:

• *Mild chronic asthma:* Intermittent and brief (less than one hour) episodes of wheezing, coughing, shortness of breath or chest tightness up to two times a week, with none of these symptoms between attacks; asthma symptoms for less than a half-hour during exercise; two or fewer episodes of nocturnal asthma or nighttime wheezing per month.

• *Moderate chronic asthma:* Asthma symptoms up to two times weekly, with exacerbations that may last several days; occasional emergency care.

• *Severe chronic asthma:* Ever-present asthma symptoms and frequent attacks; frequent episodes of nocturnal asthma; limited activity levels; occasional hospitalization and emergency treatment.

Q: How is this new classification system used?

A: The distinctions between intermittent asthma and the levels of chronic asthma are particularly useful to physicians and pharmacists when prescribing asthma medications. We discuss pharmaceutical treatment in Chapter 4.

Q: Are asthma attacks predictable?

A: If you have a known trigger, you can be pretty sure that your airways will react unless you are able to counter the effects of the trigger with medication or other appropriate self-care. But, in general, asthma attacks are notoriously unpredictable. You don't know when an attack may come on; nor can you forecast its intensity or its length.

Q: Why do some asthma attacks last longer than others?

A: Part of the answer lies in airway inflammation—that asthmatic response that makes the bronchial walls swollen and puffy. A bronchospasm may resolve in a matter of minutes, but the effects of inflammation may take days or weeks to pass. Inflammation puts the asthmatic person at risk of more frequent attacks as time goes on.

Q: You talked briefly about inflammation earlier, but I'm still a little confused. What causes this inflammation?

A: One current theory links inflammation to the body's immune system, which is overactive in a person with asthma. When asthma triggers are inhaled, the immune system releases **immunoglobulins**, or protein antibodies, which attach themselves to **mast cells** found throughout the bronchial tree. The immunoglobulins attack and combine with the inhaled trigger, and the mast cells take this as a signal to release inflammatory chemicals called **mediators** into the tissues lining the nose and airway. The mediators provoke swelling and inflammation and sometimes propel mucus production and bronchospasms. One mediator that you've no doubt heard of is histamine, which we talk about in Chapter 2. There are many other mediators—as there are other theories to explain the origin of inflammation.

Q: And this inflammation is a problem because . . . ?

A: Because it can increase the severity of an asthmatic episode. If airways are already narrowed because of inflammation, then any other airway narrowing—caused by bronchospasms or mucus production—will worsen the attack. Today, researchers believe that inflammation is a key factor influencing the frequency and severity of asthma attacks.

Q: How long does the inflammation last?

A: Unlike bronchospasms, which occur over a relatively short time span and then go away, airway inflammation tends to linger. Recent research suggests that people with asthma may have low-level inflammation in the bronchial passageway for months or years after a severe attack. And as we mentioned earlier, researchers have uncovered recent evidence that inflammation is present in most asthma, even mild cases.

Inflammation can make it difficult to tell when one asthma attack ends and the next one begins: Sometimes what a person thinks represents a second attack is actually a continuation of the first.

Q: How can that be?

A: In general, a person with asthma experiences difficulties shortly after being exposed to an allergen or irritant. This is called an **immediate reaction**, and it takes place within 15 to 30 minutes of exposure. In an hour or two, once the symptoms are under control, normal breathing resumes. Everyone assumes the attack is over—and for many asthmatic people, it is. However, in approximately half of people with asthma, the attack will once again worsen 4 to 12 hours after initial exposure. The second episode will include shortness of breath, chest tightness and perhaps wheezing, and these symptoms may be more severe and longer lasting than the immediate reaction. This second episode is known as a **delayed reaction** or a **late response**.

Q: What causes a delayed response?

A: Many doctors now believe that immediate responses are caused by bronchospasms, while late responses are the result of inflammation, a hidden problem that develops slowly in the bronchial walls.

Q: Is delayed response a problem?

A: It's often disarming, because the person might assume that she is experiencing a new asthma attack, not a continuation of the first one. As a result, she might try to treat the second episode as if it were bronchospasms. However, inflammation does not respond to medications designed to treat bronchospasms. And with improper treatment, the person's asthma might continue to get worse.

Q: Can anyone have a delayed response?

A: It appears that people with extrinsic (allergic) asthma are more likely to experience late responses, and anyone who has had a delayed reaction in the past is apt to have one again. Clearly, anyone with asthma needs to determine if she is likely to have a delayed response, because that will influence what steps she'll take to control her exposure to triggers and what kind of medications she will use.

Related to inflammation is a situation that physicians call **hypersensitivity**.

Q: Which is what?

A: Hypersensitivity is what people with asthma describe as having lungs that feel "twitchy." With frequent exposure to triggers, their airways ultimately become more sensitive to all irritants. They become supersensitive and highly reactive, meaning that an asthma attack can be provoked by the slightest exposure.

Q: What happens if an attack is left untreated?

A: Sometimes nothing; some mild asthma attacks disappear on their own. As medical researchers learn more about the role of inflammation in asthma, however, they stress the need to treat even mild episodes of the disease. As we've seen, an underlying inflammation can add to airway narrowing and intensify the effect of bronchospasms or mucus production. If the inflammation spreads, it means more areas of the lung are impeded. At the very least, untreated asthma may lengthen the amount of time an asthmatic person feels miserable. At its very worst, it progresses to a severe asthma attack.

Q: How does a severe asthma attack develop?

A: A severe attack begins with the typical asthma symptoms—the ones we discussed on pages 19 and 20. As it progresses, the person under attack becomes extremely anxious and apprehensive. Flaring nostrils and bulging neck muscles are signs that breathing has become hard work. The person sweats, his breath becomes shallow, his heart beats rapidly and his blood pressure may surge up and down. Shallow inhalations become more rapid—a situation called *hyperventilation*—as air gets trapped in the lungs. The lungs may become overinflated.

Eventually, too much air is trapped in the lungs, and carbon dioxide begins to build up there. The person develops **cyanosis**—a bluish-purplish tint to the skin, particularly around the lips—which indicates insufficient oxygen in the blood. Lung function deteriorates, wheezing diminishes ("silent lung") and the sufferer becomes speechless, exhausted and confused.

Acute severe asthma and **status asthmaticus** are the medical terms for this sudden, serious attack, which the person's usual medication is powerless to control. Status asthmaticus can be fatal. Immediate emergency treatment is vital.

Q: Does status asthmaticus develop quickly?

A: It may take hours, but all too often it comes on suddenly and maybe not in the particular order we just listed. Sometimes the entire process happens in a matter of minutes. The clue that a problem is developing is the failure of usual medications to control the attack. When that happens, additional medical treatment is needed.

Q: Can a severe attack permanently damage the lungs?

A: Earlier we mentioned that asthma is a reversible disease. Because asthma is reversible, it means that asthma attacks do not lead to permanent damage in the lungs, except in rare cases. Once bronchospasms have passed, mucus production has slowed and inflammation has gone down, the lungs again operate efficiently.

Q: You mentioned that asthma deaths are preventable. How?

A: Experts believe that most asthma deaths—close to 90 percent of them—are preventable. Death can take place when the asthma sufferer and his doctor fail to recognize the severity or the speed of the attack, and thus the asthmatic person doesn't get effective medical treatment. Other factors contributing to avoidable deaths include the failure to closely monitor a hospitalized asthmatic person and the inappropriate prescription of drugs and sedatives. (Sedatives inhibit the lungs' function and should never be used during an asthma attack.) Obviously, the key to preventing asthma-related death is better medical care. We'll discuss this very important factor later in this book.

Q: Is there a profile of the person who may be at risk?

A: Researchers have linked numerous factors to an increased risk of asthma-related death. Risk factors include a history of acute severe asthma and hospitalization; lack of adequate and ongoing medical care with preventive and follow-up therapy; complacency or underestimation of the disease's severity—underestimations by the person with asthma, his family, his physician or his hospital. Issues of race and poverty also play a role: Among African Americans the asthma death rate is almost three times higher than among Caucasians. In younger age-groups—15 to 44 years of age—the death rates for African Americans are nearly five times higher, particularly in urban centers.

All that said, we have some very reassuring news.

Q: Which is . . . ?

A: Few asthma attacks are life-threatening, even those that require some emergency-room or hospital care. In fact, most people with asthma can live normal, active lives with few restrictions. By understanding the disease, controlling triggers, practicing sound self-care and forging a partnership with a health-care practitioner, someone with asthma need never experience a life-threatening attack. We talk about these points in the next chapters.

2 ASTHMA TRIGGERS

Q: How many asthma triggers exist?

A: There are hundreds of asthma triggers. In one person or another, almost any inhaled substance can cause the chemical reactions in the lungs that lead to the three elements of an asthma attack: bronchospasms, inflammation and excessive mucus production. At any one time, the person with asthma may have several triggers activating her asthma.

Q: Where are triggers found?

A: Triggers can be found in the house, school, workplace and outdoor environment.

Q: Okay, there are hundreds of triggers. But are some triggers more common than others?

A: Yes. Over the years, asthmatic people and their doctors have discovered that certain substances provoke asthma attacks. The substances range from allergens, chemical irritants, air pollutants and tobacco smoke to food intolerances and drug sensitivities. Certain situations are also linked with asthma flare-ups: exercise, infections, stress and weather patterns.

For children and adults with extrinsic, or allergic, asthma, the most common triggers are allergens.

Q: Again, an allergen is . . . ?

A: Any substance to which someone is allergic. Allergens trigger extrinsic asthma by causing the body's immune system to produce an antibody called **immunoglobulin E**, or **IgE**. When IgE comes in contact with an allergen, strong chemicals (called mediators) are released. One of these mediators, histamine, produces an allergic reaction. In a person with extrinsic asthma, the reaction displays itself in the form of asthma symptoms.

Q: Can you give an example of these allergens?

A: Many allergens are found in household dust, including pollen, mold, animal dander and dust mites. Small in size, these allergens are easily stirred up, carried in the air and then inhaled; for that reason they are also known as **aeroallergens**. Let's take a closer look at the common aeroallergens.

POLLEN

Q: What is pollen?

A: This is a tiny grain or granule produced by trees, grasses, weeds and flowers as part of the plant world's reproductive process. Each plant or tree can be a prolific source of pollen, producing hundreds of pollen grains every year.

Some pollens are extremely lightweight and are carried by the wind for up to several hundred miles. Grass, ragweed and tree pollens tend to fall into this category. Other pollens, such as those of goldenrod and many hybrid flowers, are heavier and must be carried by insects.

Q: Is one form of pollen more bothersome?

A: As one might expect, lightweight pollens pose a greater threat to those allergic to them. Lightweight pollen drifts easily into the house, workplace or automobile through open doors and windows, where the pollen becomes part of household dust. A single open window can be the source of pollen throughout an entire house!

Q: Isn't pollen just a problem in spring?

A: Depending upon what region of the country you live in, pollen may be a problem from spring until the first killing frost. It may be present 6 to 12 months of the year. As a rule of thumb, trees pollinate in spring, grasses in summer and ragweed in late summer and fall.

Pollen allergies are more active on dry, windy days. Rain causes pollen to settle to the ground, thus temporarily lowering pollen levels out-of-doors.

MOLD SPORES

Q: What is a mold spore?

A: Mold, also called mildew or fungus, is a living organism that reproduces by producing microscopic spores that float through the air. These spores, not the parent mold, cause asthma symptoms.

Molds love humidity, and indoors they flourish year-round in bathrooms, kitchens, closets and basements—any place with humidity levels above 50 percent. Refrigerators can harbor molds, as can humidifiers, water vaporizers and air conditioners. Elsewhere in the home lurk other trouble spots: shower curtains, bathroom tiles and sweaty toilets; old mattresses, foam pillows and stuffed animals; the leaves and soil of potted plants; even old newspapers. Some foods, such as beer and many cheeses, contain mold.

Mold and fungi proliferate outdoors too, on compost piles, leaves, mulches, plants and in the soil itself. They grow with vigor when the weather is warm and moist.

ANIMAL DANDER AND SALIVA

Q: What is animal dander?

A: Dander refers to tiny pieces of sloughed-off skin (much like human dandruff) from warm-blooded animals: cats, dogs, horses, birds and rodents. People who have pets certainly will have animal dander in their home environments. The tiny flakes or scales easily become airborne and become part of house dust, remaining in a room long after the pet has left it. Zoos, farms and stables are other places where animal dander can be found. When inhaled by a person who is allergic to it, dander triggers asthma symptoms.

Q: Why is animal saliva a problem?

A: When an animal licks its fur, it covers its hair with saliva. Particles of dried saliva are shed with the hair and eventually make their way into the dust that moves through the air and settles on every exposed surface in a room. As with dander, the saliva particles are inhaled and activate the cycle of asthmatic symptoms. The cause of this reaction appears to be a particular protein in saliva. More people are allergic to cats than any other animal, simply because cats are fastidious groomers and lick their fur frequently.

Q: Can people be allergic to animal hair?

A: Most experts agree that the hair itself is not the problem. Instead, the dander and saliva associated with animal fur act as the triggers.

DUST MITES

Q: What are these?

A: Also called house-dust mites, these are microscopic creatures that feed on sloughed-off flakes of human skin. They live in carpets, mattresses and pillows, upholstered furniture and other household fabrics. Any place where humans congregate, mites may be present.

Dust mites are prolific, laying 50 eggs every 10 days or so, according to some estimates. The allergic reaction comes not from the live mite but from contact with insect debris—fecal particles and decomposed body parts—that becomes part of airborne household dust.

Q: Are dust mites found throughout the United States?

A: To thrive, mites need humidity levels above 50 percent. Most parts of the country have moisture levels that high for a portion of the year—summer in particular. People have dust mites in their homes during humid periods unless those homes are kept very dry. Mites are less of a problem in cold, dry winter months.

Q: If I move to a dry climate, will my home be mite-free?

A: People who live in dry climates are not necessarily out of the woods: They may inadvertently create a breeding ground for dust mites if they use a humidifier to bring moisture levels above 50 percent.

COCKROACHES

Q: You mean to say that people are allergic to roaches?

A: Yes. In the same way that they can be allergic to dust-mite debris, asthmatic people can be allergic to cockroach debris—fecal particles and decomposed body parts.

Q: I've never heard of this allergy before. Is it common?

A: Until the 1990s, a cockroach was not generally thought of as an asthma trigger. But as medical researchers looked to explain increasing asthma mortality in

American cities, they discovered that many city dwellers had
a cockroach allergy.

   In one study reported in *Medical World News*, cockroach
allergy was found in over one-third of the asthmatic inner-
city residents surveyed. Cockroaches are not thought to be a
large factor in asthma in suburban America, however.

Q: Are there similar triggers I should be aware of?

A: The aeroallergens we've just discussed are the most
common triggers of extrinsic asthma. But there are
also a large number of nonallergic triggers that medical practitioners refer to as *asthma irritants*. They provoke the lungs
of people with the intrinsic, or nonallergic, form of asthma.

Q: How do irritants differ from allergens?

A: Irritants, as their name implies, provoke an asthma
attack by irritating the lungs and starting the cycle of
bronchospasms, mucus production and airway inflammation.
Allergens cause immunoglobulin E and mast cells to release
histamine and other mediators; irritants do not trigger this
allergic process.

   Let's look at some of the more common irritants.

CHEMICALS

Q: How can chemicals trigger asthma?

A: Common household chemicals and personal-care
products can trigger asthma symptoms by producing

aerosols and gases that irritate the lungs. These are known as airborne chemical irritants.

Q: Which chemicals act as airborne irritants?

A: Spray disinfectants, ammonia, chlorine, floor wax and paint; perfumes, powders, deodorants, shampoos and hair sprays; and pesticides and insecticides (particularly those containing pyrethrum). The propellants and dispersants in some antiasthma medications can actually cause a chronic asthma-related cough. Even cooking odors can trigger asthma symptoms.

Airborne chemical irritants can come in unexpected packages. A report in a 1993 issue of *American Family Physician* warned that the deployment of automobile airbags can cause breathing problems for people with asthma. The problem appears not to be caused by the chemicals that fill the airbag, but by chemicals produced when the airbag is deployed.

Q: What about chemicals in the environment?

A: They too can cause problems, particularly in the form of air pollution.

AIR POLLUTANTS

Q: Which pollutants cause asthma?

A: Asthma is aggravated by irritants that are by-products of the industrialized world in which we live. Sulfur dioxide, diesel-fuel exhaust, automobile exhaust and emission plumes from factories and incinerators are among the offenders. Brushfires, burning leaves and burning garbage also release irritating particles into the air. Smog can trigger an asthma attack. So too can fog, by carrying air pollutants as an easily inhaled mist.

Q: Is it better for someone with asthma to live in the countryside?

A: Pollutants are found in major metropolitan and industrial areas, but the countryside is not necessarily pollution-free. The wind carries many pollutants to rural communities far from the city. Remember, too, that pollen is a major trigger, and pollen-producing plants grow in abundance in the countryside.

Q: What's this I hear about pollution and ozone?

A: Formed by a photochemical reaction of sunlight on already particle-laden air, ozone is a major lower-atmosphere pollutant. (In the upper layers of the atmosphere, it protects our planet from ultraviolet radiation.) While ozone can irritate the airways of someone without asthma, its debilitating effects are multiplied in the lungs of people with asthma.

TOBACCO SMOKE

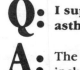

Q: I suppose you're going to say that people with asthma shouldn't smoke?

A: The evidence speaks for itself. Tobacco smoke—including cigarette, pipe and cigar smoke—is a major

indoor pollutant and an irritant that creates breathing difficulties in the lungs of any asthmatic person who smokes. There
is also increasing evidence that passive smoking—exposure
to secondhand smoke—leads to more-frequent respiratory
problems among asthmatic children and more-frequent and
severe asthma episodes among asthmatic older people.

Q: Why does smoke cause problems?

A: Tobacco smoke contains carbon monoxide, nicotine
and other harmful substances that damage the **cilia**,
delicate hairlike structures in the airways that help filter air
and clear out mucus. The longer someone is exposed to
tobacco smoke, the more damage to his cilia. With the cilia
unable to work properly, inhaled particles begin to build up
in and obstruct his air passages. Asthma attacks and respiratory infections can follow—not to mention an increased risk
of developing lung cancer and other diseases associated with
smoke inhalation.

Q: Are other kinds of smoke a problem?

A: You've raised a good point. The by-products of any
kind of fire or combustion can be irritants. Earlier
we mentioned brushfires and burning leaves. Other irritating
smoke and gases can build up in the air when natural gas or
kerosene is burned in the home without adequate ventilation,
or when poorly sealed wood stoves or fireplaces are used to
burn wood.

OCCUPATIONAL TRIGGERS

Q: What are these—triggers that occur at work?

A: Occupational triggers are irritating substances in the workplace that lead to what is called **occupational asthma**. This is asthma that develops from repeated exposure to large amounts of one particular substance found at a job site. Once a person has become sensitized to the substance (which may be an allergen or an irritant), even the slightest exposure to the substance sets off bronchoconstriction.

For example, bakers exposed to vast amounts of flour all day may develop asthmatic symptoms whenever they come in contact with flour. Meat wrappers experience reactions from inhaling polyvinyl chloride fumes from plastic wrap. Farmers, welders, carpenters, painters, plastics workers and people in the pharmaceutical industry are among the dozens of people with documented cases of occupational asthma.

Q: How many people have occupational asthma?

A: Researchers estimate that 2 percent of all asthma may be caused by exposure to a sensitizing substance at the worksite. While occupational asthma is not always an allergic response, some physicians believe that people with allergies are at greater risk of developing it. Occupational asthma and its triggers are difficult to detect, particularly if the person experiences a delayed response to an offending substance. One sign of occupational asthma is the absence of symptoms when away from the job site, such as during weekends or vacations.

Q: But a person's occupation is her livelihood—
if someone has occupational asthma, will she
have to find other work?

A: In some cases, yes. Occupational asthma differs from
other forms of asthma in one important respect: It is
not always reversible, meaning that medications may cease to
prevent or contain asthma attacks. If that happens, eliminating
exposure to the irritating substance is the recommended
treatment, even if that means changing jobs.

ADVERSE FOOD REACTIONS

Q: Can what I eat cause asthma attacks?

A: Some people have allergies to certain foods or
intolerances to food additives. These *adverse food
reactions*, as allergists term them, can provoke severe or even
life-threatening asthma attacks.

Some adverse food reactions are allergic: When an offending food is eaten, the immune system kicks into action,
releasing immunoglobulin E to attack and interact with the
allergen in the food. The mast cells then release histamine
and other mediators, which cause allergic and asthmatic
symptoms. Typical food allergens for children include eggs,
milk, wheat, corn, peanuts, soy, shellfish, citrus juices, arti-
ficial coloring and some flavorings. Adults tend to be allergic
to peanuts, tree nuts, eggs, yeast products, shellfish and fish.

The good news for youngsters is that allergies to milk,
wheat, eggs and corn are often outgrown. However, allergies
to fish, shellfish, nuts and peanuts tend to remain for life,
and the severity of reactions to these lifelong allergens often
increases with each exposure.

Q: You mentioned food intolerances.
What are they?

A: Food intolerances are nonallergic food reactions.
Something in the food causes the mast cells to release
mediators, but the process is not a result of an interaction
between IgE antibodies and allergens. In short, the "mechanism" may be different from a food allergy, but the resulting
symptoms are the same.

Q: What is the most common food intolerance?

A: The intolerance to **sulfites**, chemical preservatives
used on fruits and vegetables, in wine and in drugs
to retard spoilage. Sulfites can cause severe and even fatal
asthma episodes. Although the Food and Drug Administration
has banned the use of sulfites on fresh fruits and vegetables,
sulfites are found in some processed potatoes, dried fruits,
shrimp, beer and wine. Sulfites are also used as preservatives
in some asthma medications! Isoethrine (a bronchodilator
sold under the name of Bronkosol), a corticosteroid by the
name of Solucortef and epinephrine (Adrenalin) are three
such drugs. We'll talk about these drugs in Chapter 4.

DRUG SENSITIVITIES

Q: Which drugs trigger asthma?

A: According to the National Asthma Education Program,
5 to 20 percent of asthmatic adults experience severe
and even fatal asthma attacks after taking aspirin or certain
other nonsteroidal anti-inflammatory drugs. Someone with
severe asthma is more likely to experience such problems
than someone with mild asthma. Many people with aspirin

sensitivity also have **nasal polyps**, grapelike protrusions in the lining of the nose. (We'll discuss nasal polyps in a moment.)

Because of this, asthma experts advise that people with asthma avoid aspirin and other nonsteroidal anti-inflammatory medications. These include ibuprofen (Motrin, Advil, Nuprin), naproxen (Naprosyn, Anaprox) and piroxican. Your doctor can direct you to a safe alternative, which may include acetaminophen, sodium salicylate or disalcid.

Q: Do other drugs cause asthma attacks?

A: One possible drug is tartrazine (yellow food dye #5), used in food and medicine. It has been linked with occurrences of acute bronchoconstriction, but rarely. In addition, beta blockers—drugs designed to lower high blood pressure—can trigger bronchoconstriction. People with asthma are generally advised not to take them. Finally, be aware that many medications can produce adverse reactions when taken in combination with asthma drugs. Your doctor should give you information on possible drug interactions.

EXERCISE

Q: Is exercise an irritant?

A: Yes. As we saw in Chapter 1, exercise can trigger bronchospasms, which lead to shortness of breath, chest pain or tightness, wheezing, coughing or endurance problems during vigorous exercise. Exercise-induced asthma is very common in people of all ages. The bronchospasms may come on a few minutes after exercise starts, peak 5 to 10 minutes after the vigorous activity stops, and disappear 20, 30 or 60 minutes later. The more intense the exercise, the more severe the attack.

For some people, exercise is the only trigger for asthma. These episodes may occur only during cold weather, although some asthmatic people experience exercise-induced asthma all year round. Sexual intercourse can be a cause of exercise-induced asthma.

INFECTIONS

Q: What kinds of infections trigger asthma?

A: Viral respiratory infections, such as the common cold and influenza, and bacterial respiratory infections are two culprits. Children and adults are equally vulnerable.

Q: Do colds often trigger asthma?

A: Definitely. A study of men and women with asthma noted that colds were reported in 80 percent of episodes of wheezing, chest tightness or breathlessness, and that 89 percent of colds were associated with asthma symptoms (*British Medical Journal*, October 16, 1993).

People with asthma notice that once colds develop, they tend to linger. Doctors aren't sure why this happens. Some suggest that certain viruses make the lungs more irritable, thus setting the stage for an attack. Others say that the increased mucus production of a cold, on top of the asthmatic lung's already high production of mucus, pushes the asthmatic person's respiratory system over the edge.

Q: What about bacterial infections?

A: These include infections such as **pneumonia** and strep throat. Bacterial infections may follow as a complication of a common cold. They may develop in the area around a mucus plug that the person with asthma has been unable to dislodge.

Q: Is a sinus infection a problem, too?

A: Indeed, yes. Known in medical parlance as **sinusitis**, it is an inflammation of the mucous membrane of the sinuses—the open cavities in the head behind the nose and eyes. Swelling and inflammation there may eventually affect the bronchial tubes and worsen asthma.

Sinusitis may be caused by a viral or a bacterial infection. Often it starts as a common cold that later develops into a secondary bacterial infection. Symptoms include headache, sinus tenderness, nausea, postnasal drip, fever and a yellowish or greenish discharge from the nose. While sinusitis persists, asthma symptoms are difficult—if not impossible—to control.

WEATHER

Q: How does weather trigger asthma?

A: Sudden changes in weather fronts or barometric pressure are associated with the worsening of asthma, for reasons that are unclear.

Many people report asthma problems on cold winter days, possibly because dry, frigid air is a shock to the sensitive bronchial passageways. Warm, humid days prove problematic, too, in part because mold and pollen grow when humidity is high. A strong wind may blow pollutants away or it may bring in fresh batches of pollen from afar. Rain may settle dust and pollen and give the allergic asthmatic person a measure of relief, or rain may encourage the growth of mold.

STRESS

Q: Didn't you already say that stress doesn't cause asthma?

A: Emotions and stress do not cause asthma in someone who does not already have the disease. However, stress and other emotions, such as anxiety and anger, do increase the frequency and intensity of asthma attacks.

That may be because strong emotions affect people in obvious physical ways: People tense their muscles in highly charged situations; some hyperventilate or pant in response to stress. This doesn't explain the full link between emotions and asthma, but it does point to the usefulness of breathing and relaxation exercises and other techniques for stress control. You'll find details about these in Chapter 5.

Exercise, infections, weather and stress are all situations that can lead to or intensify an asthma attack. Now let's turn our attention in another direction, toward *medical conditions* that can worsen asthma.

Q: Which medical conditions make asthma worse?

A: For starters, **allergic rhinitis** (commonly called hay fever) makes asthma more difficult to control. Like extrinsic asthma, allergic rhinitis is an allergic response to an inhaled substance (the allergen). In asthma this response occurs in the bronchial tree; in allergic rhinitis, the reaction takes place in the eyes, nose and throat, usually in the form of watery eyes, congestion, runny nose, sneezing, scratchy throat and coughing.

Q: **How does hay fever affect asthma?**

A: The congestion and throat irritation seen in hay fever may reach the lungs, causing bronchial inflammation and provoking an asthma attack. Allergic rhinitis and asthma often operate in tandem: People with asthma may develop allergic rhinitis (particularly if they are under age 40), just as someone with hay fever may one day develop asthma.

People with allergic rhinitis tend to have asthma problems for an additional reason—they develop nasal polyps.

Q: **What are these?**

A: When the cells of the mucous membrane lining the nose produce too much fluid, that area of the membrane stretches and protrudes into the nasal cavity. These fluid-filled, grapelike protrusions are known as nasal polyps. Although they are in themselves harmless, they can block nasal passageways and make breathing difficult.

One important fact to know is that asthmatic people with nasal polyps tend to be extremely allergic to aspirin. They are advised to avoid any aspirin-containing products.

Doctors frequently prescribe medicated nasal sprays to treat nasal polyps. Surgery is sometimes recommended, although nasal polyps tend to reappear, even after surgery.

Q: Are there other conditions related to asthma?

A: Another is **gastroesophageal reflux**—the regurgitation of stomach acids into the esophagus. Sometimes this process is called acid reflux; you and I know it as heartburn.

Q: What causes this?

A: It happens when the muscle valve between the esophagus and the stomach fails to seal tightly. Acidic contents from the stomach travel up into the esophagus or even into the pharynx, resulting in belching and the sensation of heartburn. If someone with asthma inhales this acidic material into the larynx or bronchi, bronchospasms and airway inflammation may develop.

Q: Is gastroesophageal reflux common?

A: Gastroesophageal reflux is three times more common in both children and adults with asthma than in people who do not have asthma. Doctors do not know why it occurs this frequently.

Reflux is more troublesome when an asthmatic person is reclining. Thus, it's a particular problem at night, when people with asthma are already prone to experience asthma problems.

Q: How is it treated?

A: If you have this problem, your doctor may advise you to eat smaller but more frequent meals; avoid food or drink between dinner and bedtime; and avoid fatty meals, spices and alcohol. Elevating the head of your bed may help, too. Some medications used in treating asthma, such as theophylline (which we discuss in Chapter 4), may make reflux worse. Surgery is sometimes recommended, but it's not always successful.

Q: We've discussed allergens, irritants and conditions that worsen asthma. Are there any other triggers?

A: As we mentioned at the start of this chapter, there are hundreds of asthma triggers. Some triggers may still be unknown. The key points are to realize that many substances can cause asthma attacks and to take steps to discover which ones affect you.

3 TESTS AND PROCEDURES

Q: How important is it that asthma be diagnosed early?

A: The sooner you get a handle on *any* disease, the sooner you can gain control over your health. Because asthma interferes with the process by which oxygen is delivered to the body's cells, it is important to address asthma and the associated breathing difficulties promptly.

That said, people with asthma have an advantage in that asthma is a controllable disease. In all but the rarest, most extreme cases, asthma can be controlled—even to the point that it appears to go away—no matter at what stage the disease is diagnosed.

Q: Where does one begin in diagnosing asthma?

A: The first matter of business is distinguishing asthma from so-called similar conditions.

Q: Again, those similar conditions are . . . ?

A: If a child swallows an object that lodges in the throat or air passages, airway obstruction and wheezing could result. Other causes of obstruction and wheezing in youngsters are infections, viral **bronchiolitis** (an inflammation of the lining of the bronchioles that obstructs the passage of air) or cystic fibrosis.

In adults, causes might include chronic bronchitis, emphysema, heart failure, a blood clot in the lungs (known as a **pulmonary embolism**), a growth of mold spores in the air passages (known as **allergic bronchopulmonary aspergillosis**), a problem in the larynx, or a reaction to a drug, such as a beta blocker.

Q: How do doctors distinguish these conditions from asthma?

A: Doctors generally take a person's medical history, perform a physical examination and evaluate his or her pulmonary function (medical lingo for how well the lungs operate). Doctors look for two signposts of asthma: first, that airway obstruction or narrowing is episodic, and second, that airway obstruction improves with medication or other self-care. Tests and procedures may be ordered to rule out other causes of airway obstruction or to detect the presence of another medical condition.

Q: What is a medical history?

A: It is a compilation of information about a person's health and is based in large part on questions that a doctor poses to the medical consumer during an initial consultation. In fact, when compiling a medical history, the doctor should ask questions and do the listening; the medical consumer is the one who should do the talking.

Q: **What sorts of questions?**

A: The following are among questions the physician
may ask. And if she doesn't ask them, the patient
certainly can volunteer the information.

The practitioner may begin by asking for a description of
symptoms and the pattern in which symptoms occur. Are
symptoms present seasonally or year-round? daily or occasionally? during the day or at night? at home or at work? more
common indoors or outdoors? The patient may follow with
a description of a typical flare-up of symptoms (how it begins
and progresses, how he treats it and how it usually ends).

The patient should point out the situations that make
symptoms worse. Do flare-ups accompany respiratory infections, exposure to allergens, irritants or certain foods, exercise,
strong emotions, drugs, weather changes or other triggers
discussed in Chapter 2? If the person thought to have asthma
is an infant, do feedings, position or excitement worsen
symptoms? What is the person's occupation or, in the case
of a child, what are the parents' occupations?

Home environment is another topic of discussion. Is the
home old or new? heated with oil, gas, electricity, coal, kerosene or wood? Does the home have high humidity levels? a
damp basement? carpeting over a concrete slab floor? Is
there a pet in the house? a cigarette smoker? What sorts of
dust collectors are found in the asthmatic person's bedroom?

Q: **Is this the right time to discuss the health
of other family members?**

A: Absolutely. One part of the discussion should determine whether any family members have allergies or
asthma. Another part should focus on the patient's own
symptom history, including his age at onset of symptoms,
whether symptoms have gotten better or worse, how they
have been treated in the past and present, whether he has
other allergies or conditions that make asthma worse, and
whether he smokes cigarettes.

It's also helpful to discuss the impact of symptoms on everyday life. How many school or workdays have been missed? Do symptoms limit activity, particularly sports? How many urgent-care visits have been made to a doctor's office or emergency room? Has the person ever been hospitalized for life-threatening attacks? How do asthma problems affect the rest of his family? Can family members distinguish between a mild flare-up and a serious one? Do the symptomatic person and his family feel equipped to cope with the disease?

With responses to these and other questions, a doctor may be able to surmise that asthma is present.

Q: **What if the patient is a child with a very limited medical history?**

A: Diagnosing a young child with chronic or recurring episodes of coughing or wheezing is something of a challenge, doctors admit. When medical history is limited, the physical examination and basic laboratory tests take on more importance.

Q: **Let's talk about the patient's physical exam. What does it entail?**

A: In both adults and children, the doctor will focus on the upper respiratory tract, the chest and the skin. She will look for the presence of hay fever, sinus infection and nasal polyps. She will listen for wheezing (the characteristic breath sound of asthma) or for long, slow, forced expiration (a sign of airflow obstruction). Skin problems, such as eczema, may signal an allergic predisposition. Cyanosis, a purple-blue skin tint in the fingertips or lips, indicates that the person is not getting enough oxygen.

In a child, the doctor will look for the appearance of hunched shoulders, malformation of the chest and other evidence that he is using other chest muscles to help his lungs push air out of narrowed passageways.

Q: **Once the medical history and physical exam are complete, can the doctor make a diagnosis of asthma?**

A: Many times, yes. In other cases, more information is needed—and this information comes from diagnostic tests and procedures.

In fact, most practitioners want to order at least a few tests and procedures to corroborate a diagnosis, rule out or locate coexisting diseases and assess asthma's severity. As a medical consumer, you should understand the purpose of any tests you or your family members are asked to take. If not, speak up. As David Tinkelman, M.D., writes in *Understanding Asthma:* "There should be a good reason for performing the tests and you should know what it is."

Q: What sorts of tests are we talking about?

A: Let's look at the first tests given to people with asthma: **pulmonary-function tests**.

PULMONARY-FUNCTION TESTS

Q: What are these?

A: Pulmonary-function tests check the dynamics of breathing. They determine how well the lungs are performing and estimate severity of airway obstruction.

Q: How are pulmonary-function tests performed?

A: They are usually done in a doctor's office or hospital on a computerized instrument called a **spirometer**. A person puts on nose clips, inhales fully and then exhales as hard as possible into a mouthpiece and tube attached to the spirometer. The instrument measures the volume of air in the lungs during exhalation (known as **lung volume measurements**) and the speed with which that air is expelled (known as **ventilation measurements**).

Four tests are done on the spirometer.

Q: And they are ... ?

A: One of the most common is the **forced expiratory volume in 1 second** or FEV_1, which measures the greatest amount of air that can be expelled in one second when the person exhales as hard as possible.

The **forced vital capacity (FVC)** test measures the total amount of air that can be exhaled as rapidly as possible, and the **maximum midexpiratory flow rate (MMEF)** shows how flow rate decreases between 25 and 75 percent of the forced expiratory volume.

Q: What is the fourth test?

A: The **peak expiratory flow rate (PEFR)**, commonly called the peak flow, measures the maximum speed at which air can leave the lungs. For this test to be accurate, the person must take a deep breath and exhale with as much energy as she can muster.

Peak-flow measurements can also be made by using a portable device, appropriately called the **peak flow meter**. As the person exhales forcefully into the mouthpiece of this tube-shaped device, an indicator scale measures the greatest speed of air leaving the lungs.

Q: Are all four pulmonary-function tests suitable for people of all ages?

A: They can be done by adults and children over age three.

Q: How are pulmonary-function measurements used?

A: After the person has done three pulmonary-function tests in a row, she takes the highest reading and compares it to a "predicted value" chart, which lists average readings arranged in categories according to age and height. A "normal" reading is one that ranges from 80 to 120 percent of the predicted value for someone in the same age-and-height category.

Q: If the readings are normal, does that rule out asthma?

A: Not necessarily. It may mean that the person is not experiencing an asthma flare-up at the moment the readings are taken. For that reason, it's a good idea to schedule an office visit during a time when asthma symptoms are evident.

REVERSIBILITY TEST

Q: What does this test achieve?

A: The reversibility test is really a pulmonary-function test performed after the patient takes a medication—usually a **bronchodilator**, an asthma drug that opens the airways. If a pulmonary-function test shows improved airflow after medication is taken, then the obstruction is considered reversible and the diagnosis of asthma is made.

Severe airflow obstruction may not immediately improve with a bronchodilator, so the physician may put the person on bronchodilators and anti-inflammatory drugs for several weeks. The test is done again. If readings improve, asthma is the likely diagnosis.

SWEAT TEST

Q: What is a **sweat test** and when is it used?

A: This simple test is administered to check for cystic fibrosis, a hereditary lung and pancreatic disease found predominantly in children. Youngsters with cystic fibrosis have more salt in their sweat than children without the disease. By collecting a small amount of sweat and analyzing its salt content, a health-care practitioner can detect or rule out cystic fibrosis in a matter of hours.

X-RAYS

Q: What **x-rays** are used to detect asthma?

A: Most physicians hold that a chest x-ray is critical to rule out other causes of airway obstruction. The chest x-ray can also disclose what parts of the lungs are obstructed and show whether mucus plugs have caused airless pockets in the lungs (a condition known as **atelectasis**). The x-ray can serve as a baseline from which to evaluate changes in the lungs' condition.

Q: Are other x-rays used?

A: Some practitioners may order a sinus x-ray to diagnose sinus infection or inflammation that could worsen asthma. Sinus x-rays are less effective in detecting problems in small children, particularly those under a year old, because their sinus cavities are not yet fully developed.

SKIN TESTS

Q: When are **skin tests** conducted?

A: Skin tests are used to determine which substances, if any, cause sensitivities or allergies.

Q: How do skin tests work?

A: There are three types of skin tests: In the **scratch test**, the doctor makes a series of short, superficial scratches on the skin, usually the forearm. Into each scratch the doctor rubs a different extract of a suspected allergen. If in 15 to 20 minutes a red, itchy welt or **wheal** develops on a scratch, it means that the person reacted positively to that substance.

Q: And the second test is . . . ?

A: The **skin-prick test**, in which a drop of allergen extract is placed on the arm. A small needle pricks the skin under the drop. A red wheal in 15 to 20 minutes indicates a positive reaction.

Q: What is the third test?

A: In the **intradermal test**, the allergen-containing solution is injected directly into the skin. Again, the doctor watches for signs of reactions.

Q: Does the presence of a wheal mean I am allergic to that substance?

A: Maybe. Positive skin-test reactions indicate the presence of antibodies. The tests show only that your body has been exposed to a particular allergen and has been sensitized to it. However, the tests do not prove that you are presently allergic to this substance or that you would have an allergic reaction if you were exposed to it. Skin tests merely demonstrate the potential to react.

Q: I've heard that reactions to skin tests can be dangerous. Is that true?

A: In rare cases, yes. Skin tests, particularly intradermal tests, have been known to cause reactions ranging from itchy skin and flushed face to blood-pressure fluctuations, difficulty breathing and even unconsciousness. For that reason, skin tests are best done under close medical supervision, where the person can be given the drug epinephrine if problems develop.

BLOOD TESTS

Q: What kind of blood tests are used in diagnosing asthma?

A: Blood tests may include a blood scan to evaluate overall health and a complete blood count to detect the presence of **eosinophils**, specialized white blood cells that release chemicals that cause inflammation in airway tissue. Eosinophils are sometimes high in people with allergies.

An immunoglobulin test may be administered to check the body's ability to fight infection. An immune-system deficiency sometimes leads to upper respiratory infections in infants, although the problem is outgrown as the immune system matures.

Blood studies may also include a total IgE measurement to check for allergies.

Q: What does an IgE measurement show?

A: A total IgE measurement may indicate that the person has sensitivities to allergens. But it won't name names, so to speak. One test that is used to pinpoint allergens is the **radioallergosorbent test**, or RAST, which measures the amount of allergen-specific IgE antibodies in the blood.

Q: How is the RAST different from other tests?

A: The RAST is sometimes used instead of a series of skin tests. A single blood sample is drawn, and allergens such as pollens, molds, animal dander and food additives are added. When the allergens bind to antibodies in the blood, laboratory technicians can measure how much antibody is present.

The advantages of the RAST and other tests like it are that they are convenient, particularly for small children, and the patients do not experience severe adverse reactions from exposure to allergens.

Q: Are RASTs better than skin tests?

A: They may be safer. On the other hand, they are more expensive and less sensitive than skin tests. In some cases, a person with asthma will need a skin test to double-check the results of the RAST.

In addition, the value of a RAST hinges on how well the test is completed. David Tinkelman, writing in *Understanding Asthma*, notes that many laboratories that perform RASTs are plagued by poor quality control, which renders their results inaccurate. For that reason, the RAST is still considered experimental.

Q: Is there any way to be certain that a substance triggers asthma?

A: Clear proof, if proof is needed, can be achieved through **bronchoprovocation**.

BRONCHOPROVOCATION

Q: What is this?

A: Bronchoprovocation, or bronchial challenge, occurs when a person with asthma is deliberately exposed to a suspected or known allergen. This is done in the doctor's office, under medical supervision, in an attempt to provoke a mild asthma attack.

Q: Why would someone deliberately try to make asthma worse?

A: This may be done if the person's symptoms suggest asthma but there is no evidence of airflow obstruction. If bronchoprovocation causes airway obstruction and asthma symptoms, asthma is the likely diagnosis.

Naturally, the goal is to provoke a mild form of asthma, not a major attack. The resulting chest discomfort can be reversed quickly by an inhaled bronchodilator.

EXERCISE CHALLENGE

Q: Is this a form of bronchoprovocation?

A: Yes. Some people experience asthma symptoms only during exercise, and an **exercise-challenge** test is needed to make the diagnosis of asthma. In other cases an exercise challenge may be used to measure the airway's sensitivity or to gauge the effectiveness of medications or other self-care.

Q: How is this test done?

A: The person is asked to jog on a treadmill, ride an exercise bike or perform some other exercise in the doctor's office. Again, the idea is to provoke mild asthma and to measure the amount of airway obstruction. A pulmonary-function test is often used to make this measurement.

FOOD CHALLENGE

Q: Is a **food challenge** yet another type of bronchoprovocation?

A: It is a more complicated process, though the end goal is to locate food intolerances or allergies. A food-challenge test is done after skin tests and RASTs suggest that certain foods are allergens. Since the latter two tests do not prove that those foods cause allergic reactions, food challenges are needed to confirm a suspected allergy.

There are two types of food challenges. The simplest is food avoidance: removing a food from the diet and observing if asthma symptoms disappear. If so, the food is later reintroduced into the diet. If asthma symptoms recur, then doctors assume that the food is a trigger.

The second, more scientific approach is **blind testing**, in which the person is given a dose of a suspected allergen or a placebo (a harmless bland substance). "Blinding" food allows the doctor to determine whether a food really does trigger asthma. It separates the foods people *think* cause a problem from those that actually do.

Q: Are food challenges dangerous?

A: Food challenges should be done sparingly and only under medical supervision. People sometimes have strong, even life-threatening reactions to food intolerances, and medical assistance should be close at hand.

SPUTUM STAIN OR MUCUS STAIN

Q: What kind of test is this?

A: A **sputum stain** or **mucus stain** entails taking a sample of **sputum** (mucus that has been coughed up from the lungs) or mucus from the nose and examining it under a microscope. These stains are used to test for the presence of eosinophils, white blood cells that play a role in airway inflammation.

While eosinophils can be measured in a blood test, a sputum analysis may reveal other facts about the lung's condition. A sputum analysis may show mucus plugs, pieces of destroyed cells or pieces of the *aspergillus* mold that causes allergic bronchopulmonary aspergillosis.

ELECTROCARDIOGRAM

Q: Why is a heart test used in asthmatic people?

A: An **electrocardiogram** (EKG) is a recording of the heart muscle's activity that is collected by electrodes placed on the chest. It may be used to detect heart conditions that mimic asthma or to monitor the effects of certain asthma drugs in people who have both asthma and heart problems.

BRONCHOSCOPY

Q: What is a **bronchoscopy?**

A: This is an examination of the bronchi via a flexible, fiberoptic viewing tube (called an **endoscope**) that has been inserted down the throat. Occasionally a doctor performs a bronchoscopy to obtain a tiny piece of lung tissue that will be analyzed under a microscope. In rare cases, bronchoscopy is used to remove thick mucus from the lungs—mucus that the person has been unable to dislodge by cough or medication.

RHINOSCOPY

Q: What is this used for?

A: A **rhinoscopy** is an examination of the interior of the nose and sinuses made by means of an endoscope. The procedure may be used to locate an obstruction in the nose, sinuses or throat.

Q: Are there other diagnostic tests I should be aware of?

A: Your doctor may recommend a few other tests for special situations. For example, an **ultrasound scan** is sometimes used to locate fluid in the sinuses.

The important thing to remember is that there should be a good reason for any test or procedure. These diagnostic tools should be used as a complement to—not as a substitute for—the medical history and physical exam.

Q: So I've been diagnosed with asthma. What's next?

A: With the diagnosis in hand, you and your doctor can devise a treatment plan. For most people, the cornerstone of this plan will be asthma medications. We discuss pharmacological management of asthma next.

4 ASTHMA MEDICATIONS

Q: Do doctors frequently prescribe asthma medicine?

A: Yes. And they do it for two reasons: to reverse symptoms during an acute attack and to prevent the onset of attacks. Consequently, asthmatic people often take prescribed daily medications along with PRN, or as-needed, ones.

Even so-called alternative medicine, such as **homeopathy**, makes use of medication. According to Andrew Lockie in *The Family Guide to Homeopathy*, many of the drugs we discuss in this chapter are compatible with homeopathic remedies.

Q: I don't like to take drugs. Are asthma medications necessary?

A: For most people with asthma, medication is an important cornerstone of their asthma-treatment plans. And unless you are able to avoid exposure to your asthma triggers, chances are good that your doctor will recommend some form of medication. Only you and your physician can decide what is necessary in your case.

Q: What drugs might my doctor prescribe?

A: The answer depends on many factors; among them, the type of asthma experienced (such as seasonal, nocturnal and/or exercise-induced), the severity of asthma (mild, moderate or severe), the triggers and the presence of other medical conditions.

And each person's unique body chemistry plays a role. People differ in their responses to medication, and not every asthma drug works for every person. There is no one-pill-suits-all drug regimen; each person with asthma needs a custom-tailored medication plan. No drug can cure asthma, but the right medication or combination of medications may do the next best thing: make you symptom-free so you can experience a full, rewarding life.

Q: Is there any way I can minimize the amount of medication I take?

A: As we'll see in Chapter 6, self-care steps, including exercise and the eradication of triggers in the home, can work in combination with medication to help the asthmatic person control the disease. For most people with asthma, it's possible to reduce dependence on medication once asthma symptoms are under control. Even so, there may be times when an additional course of medication is crucial, such as during periods of illness or stress.

Q: How are asthma medications dispensed?

A: Asthma drugs come as pills, syrups, solutions, in aerosol canisters or as powder capsules.

Pills and syrups are taken by mouth according to package directions. Solutions are placed in a **nebulizer**, a machine that converts the solution into a fine, medicated mist that is inhaled over a four- to five-minute period. Commonly found in hospitals, nebulizers also may be used in the home if the person with asthma and his family have been well trained in filling, using and sterilizing the device. Nebulizers are used by young children, some people with severe asthma and people unable to work a **metered-dose inhaler**.

Q: What is a metered-dose inhaler?

A: It's a device that houses a small aerosol canister filed with medication. The inhaler dispenses precisely measured doses of medication as small "puffs." Inhaled medications are very common in the treatment of asthma, and most inhaled medications come in metered-dose form. Inhalers deliver these drugs directly to the lungs, where asthma problems are located. And inhalers are portable, so the person with asthma can carry them anywhere.

Q: What's the proper way to use an inhaler?

A: Specific instruction sheets come with each metered-dose inhaler. If you don't get a sheet, ask your pharmacist to give you one. Many variants of the metered-dose inhaler are on the market; be sure you know how to use the particular type you have. From time to time, ask a health-care practitioner—someone with expertise in respiratory care —to watch you use the inhaler to be sure your technique is sound. Poor technique can reduce the inhaler's effectiveness.

In general, though, you begin by shaking the inhaler and removing the cap. Place the mouthpiece either just inside or one inch in front of your open mouth. As you activate the inhaler (usually by depressing the top), inhale slowly and deeply. Hold your breath for at least 10 seconds so the medication penetrates the lower airways. If your prescription requires taking a second puff, wait at least 60 seconds to give the first dose time to spread through lung tissues.

Q: What can you tell me about the drugs themselves?

A: Asthma drugs are categorized according to what they do. The two major categories of asthma medications are bronchodilators and anti-inflammatory drugs. Other drugs are sometimes prescribed for people with asthma, although they are not asthma drugs per se. These include **mucokinetic drugs**, **antihistamines** and antibiotics.

BRONCHODILATORS

Q: You've mentioned these before. These drugs counteract bronchospasms, right?

A: Correct. When the muscles that encircle the bronchial air passages constrict—as in an asthma attack—air passages narrow. Bronchodilating drugs open the airways by relaxing constricted muscles. These drugs work faster when they are inhaled, although some bronchodilators come in pills or liquids.

Q: Are bronchodilators prescribed frequently?

A: Yes. Most people with asthma use a bronchodilator in one or more of its three forms: **sympathomimetics**, **xanthines** and **anticholinergics**.

Q: Let's start with the first one—the sympathomimetics. What are these?

A: Sympathomimetic drugs are so named because they affect the sympathetic nervous system. The most famous sympathomimetic drug, **epinephrine**, or **adrenaline** (Adrenalin, EpiPen), is rarely used in day-to-day asthma management. Epinephrine is reserved for emergencies, as we'll see in Chapter 8.

Ephedrine is another sympathomimetic drug, but is less frequently used today. Although it works quickly, ephedrine may cause shakiness and tremors. Today, doctors prefer more sophisticated drugs.

Q: Such as?

A: The sympathomimetic drugs of choice are the **beta-adrenergic agonists**, alternately called beta-adrenergic stimulants, **beta-agonists**, beta-2 agonists or beta-2 sympathomimetic agents (whew!). These drugs are "beta-2 selective"; that is, they are targeted to stimulate the beta-2 receptors in the lungs. These receptors respond by relaxing bronchial muscles and opening the airways.

Q: When are these beta-adrenergic agonists used?

A: Beta-agonists, as we'll call them, can be taken in two ways: 1) on an as-needed basis to treat asthma symptoms and to prevent exercise-induced asthma attacks, or 2) several times daily as part of a plan to control chronic asthma. When used in the latter manner, beta-agonists are taken one or two puffs at a time every 4, 6, 8 or 12 hours, depending upon the particular drug you take. Your doctor should specify the precise dosage and timing.

Q: What beta-agonists are on the market?

A: They include **albuterol** (sold as Proventil and Ventolin), most frequently used as an inhaled medication but also available as pills and formulations designed for use in a nebulizer; **bitolterol** (Tornalate), **pirbuterol** (Maxair) and **salmeterol** (Serevent), all found in metered-dose inhalers; **metaproterenol** (Alupent, Metaprel), which is available in pills, metered-dose inhalers and syrups; and **terbutaline**, which comes as a metered-dose inhaler (Brethaire), a tablet (Brethine and Bricanyl) and an injection (Bricanyl).

Two older beta-agonists, **isoetharine** (Bronkometer, Bronkosol) and **isoproterenol** (Isuprel Mistometer), are not frequently prescribed. Their effects are short—two hours or so—and they have more side effects than today's newer beta-agonists.

Q: Why so many beta-agonists?

A: For reasons that are still unclear, certain people with asthma react better to one beta-agonist than another. Often there's no way to know which is the best drug other than to try.

In addition, different forms serve different purposes. Pills and syrups are used when inflammation or mucus plugs prevent an inhaled medication from reaching all areas of the lungs.

Pharmaceutical companies continue to develop new drugs that they hope will be more effective (and more profitable!) than the older ones. The current trend is to develop beta-agonists that work longer. For example, the newest, salmeterol, is a long-acting bronchodilator that can be taken once every 12 hours.

Q: You mentioned side effects—does this mean beta-agonists are unsafe?

A: Every drug has some side effect. In the case of beta-agonists, side effects include headache, rapid heartbeat, trembling, anxiety, nausea and vomiting. These are rarely troublesome, however, and are more common when people take oral forms of the drugs—pills or syrups. Inhaled forms have fewer side effects, because the medication is delivered directly to the lungs and not to the blood. Nonetheless, oral—and sometimes even inhaled—beta-agonists may not be recommended for people with heart problems, diabetes or other medical conditions.

But to speak to your question directly: Beta-agonists may be unsafe if they are used excessively—that is, more than four times a day. In 1990 a team of New Zealand researchers reported that ongoing use of beta-agonists can make asthma worse. And a study from Canada found that asthma patients using twice the recommended daily dosage faced double the risk of a fatal or near-fatal asthma attack.

Q: **Is that because people experienced more side effects?**

A: On the contrary: Researchers theorize that although beta-agonists relieve asthma symptoms very efficiently, in actuality the drugs may mask a severe underlying inflammation.

Q: **Should I stop using beta-agonists?**

A: Absolutely not, say the experts. "We don't want people stampeding off the medicine, but they have to be much more alert as to what the side effects may be," Walter O. Spitzer, M.D., told the *New York Times* (August 8, 1991). He stressed that beta-agonists can be lifesaving if they are used cautiously—once or twice daily. That translates to no more than one aerosol canister a month. If asthma symptoms can't be handled by twice-a-day inhalation of beta-agonists, then experts advise that an anti-inflammatory drug be added to the regimen. We'll talk more about this later in the chapter.

Be aware, too, that not all doctors agree with the New Zealand and Canadian studies. Harold S. Nelson, M.D., of the National Jewish Center for Immunology and Respiratory Medicine, in Denver, states that regular use of beta-agonists is appropriate. He suggests that the Canadian study included a sicker group of asthmatic people than the asthmatic population at large, and that greater asthma problems were not due to the drugs but to the severity of illness.

Q: This is confusing. Who do I believe?

A: Although doctors try to present a united front, behind the scenes, in the medical literature, differences of opinion are common. The key is to be an informed consumer: Know both sides of the story and talk to your doctor. Together you can work out a medication plan tailored to your needs.

Q: What can you tell me about the second kind of bronchodilators, the xanthines?

A: Xanthines, or methylxanthines, include the drugs **theophylline** (Aerolate, Quibron, Respid, Slo-Bid, Theo-Dur and others) and **aminophylline**, a theophylline derivative given intravenously in emergency rooms. In the popular press, xanthines are simply referred to as theophylline.

Q: What does theophylline do?

A: Scientists aren't sure how theophylline works but they know that it relaxes bronchial muscles when given in the proper dosage. Research suggests that theophylline may reduce respiratory muscle fatigue, and the latest findings indicate that theophylline also acts as a mild anti-inflammatory drug. When used in conjunction with inhaled beta-agonists, theophylline may produce an even greater bronchodilating effect.

Q: How is theophylline used?

A: The workhorse of asthma medications for over 50 years, theophylline is primarily distributed as oral medication—pills and syrups.

Both pills and syrups are available in short-acting, intermediate-acting and sustained-release (long-acting) forms. According to Stuart H. Young, M.D., writing in *The Asthma Handbook*, short-acting forms reach maximum effectiveness after two hours and are eliminated from the body in four hours; intermediate-acting forms reach full effectiveness after four hours and are eliminated after eight hours. The long-acting form must be taken several times (usually every 12 hours) for two to three days before it builds to a therapeutic level in the blood. One dose of long-acting theophylline remains in the body 16 hours or more.

Q: Which form is best?

A: It depends entirely on the person and her asthma and the treatment regimen designed in conjunction with her doctor.

Short- or intermediate-acting medications are often prescribed for people who have mild asthma with only the occasional asthma attack, although most doctors now prefer to use beta-agonists for this situation. Sustained-release preparations may be prescribed for people who have chronic asthma with frequent attacks. Some doctors also believe long-acting forms control nocturnal asthma. However, because sustained doses take longer to kick in, they are not helpful in an acute attack; another bronchodilating drug must also be taken in that event.

Q: I've heard that theophylline can be dangerous. Is that true?

A: When theophylline is used properly, it is safe and effective. However, it is a potentially toxic drug. It has a narrow "therapeutic range."

Q: What does "therapeutic range" mean?

A: This means an asthmatic person needs a certain amount of theophylline in his bloodstream to experience any benefit. Below therapeutic levels, the drug does not work. Above therapeutic levels, however, adverse reactions occur.

Q: What are some of theophylline's side effects?

A: Even when used properly, theophylline can cause irritability, restlessness, sleeping difficulties and mild headaches. This is because theophylline is a caffeine-like substance.

The following severe side effects, known as toxic reactions, should be reported *immediately* to a doctor: nausea, vomiting or stomachache; loss of appetite; irregular heartbeat; severe headache; confusion or disorientation; seizure. Be aware that a toxic reaction to theophylline can mimic flu symptoms.

Q: How can I be sure I'm taking the proper amount of theophylline?

A: Theophylline levels are measured by blood tests. These tests are done when you start theophylline therapy and then at 6- to 12-month intervals. Blood tests may be needed if you start feeling side effects while on your usual dose, if the theophylline doesn't seem to be combating bronchospasms, or if conditions known to alter theophylline metabolism exist.

Q: What do you mean by "theophylline metabolism"?

A: We're referring to the rate at which the body breaks down theophylline. Someone whose body metabolizes theophylline quickly needs more theophylline than someone who metabolizes it slowly. As a rule, children metabolize theophylline faster than adults do, so they need more medication per pound of body weight. Smoking or exposure to cigarette smoke causes the body to burn theophylline more quickly.

Other factors can cause the body to metabolize the drug more slowly—and that's when the danger of overdose develops.

Q: And those factors are . . . ?

A: Fevers and viral infections; liver disease; heart disease; flu vaccines; and certain drugs, including the antibiotic erythromycin, oral contraceptives, ulcer drugs and a number of heart medications can all slow theophylline metabolism. A person needs less theophylline under those circumstances. Check with your doctor if any of these situations apply to you. He may tell you to cut your theophylline dose and ask you to come in for a blood test.

Q: Is it safe to use generic theophylline?

A: Different brands differ slightly in makeup and concentration. For that reason, most doctors believe it's better to stick to the same brand all the time.

Q: Using theophylline sure is complicated.
Is it worth it?

A: For the right person, theophylline is an excellent drug.
The message here is that anyone using theophylline must be alert to signs of theophylline toxicity and speak immediately to her doctor if anything seems awry. Some people cannot tolerate theophylline at therapeutic levels and thus must use other asthma drugs.

Q: Speaking of other asthma drugs, can we talk now about the third type of bronchodilator?

A: Certainly. These are the anticholinergic drugs, sometimes referred to as the **parasympatholytics** because they affect the parasympathetic nervous system. Anticholinergics open the airways and block the production of chemicals that cause bronchospasms.

The original anticholinergic, **atropine**, is now rarely prescribed; its side effects (drying of respiratory secretions, blurred vision, irregular heartbeat) outweigh its effectiveness as a bronchodilator. Today's anticholinergic of choice is **ipratropium bromide** (Atrovent), an atropine derivative that lacks atropine's side effects.

Q: What does ipratropium do?

A: Ipratropium is an inhaled bronchodilator that is slower-acting than beta-agonists, taking about an hour to reach peak effectiveness (albuterol takes five minutes) but lasting twice as long. Ipratroprium's strength appears to lie in its ability to intensify the bronchodilating effect of other asthma drugs. But there is still no medical consensus on how this drug should be used in a daily asthma medication plan.

Q: Does it have side effects?

A: A dry mouth and palpitations are the most common. Occasionally it leads to difficulty in urination and it can make glaucoma worse. But ipratropium appears to be effective against both extrinsic- and intrinsic-asthma triggers.

ANTI-INFLAMMATORY MEDICATIONS

Q: How are these drugs used in treating asthma?

A: Anti-inflammatory medications have a **prophylactic** —meaning preventive—action. They prevent inflammation in the airways or, if inflammation is already present, stop it from getting worse.

Once reserved for people with severe asthma, **anti-inflammatories** are now the first line of defense in many asthma-management programs. Experts believe that anyone with asthma who needs to take a bronchodilator daily should also be taking anti-inflammatory medication.

Q: Why is that?

A: Once airway walls are thickened by inflammation, even the slightest exposure to a trigger will set off bronchospasms, and even minor bronchospasms dramatically reduce airflow.

In contrast, people taking inhaled anti-inflammatories are less likely to respond to triggers. According to an article in *Medical Tribune* (July 9, 1992), anti-inflammatories can mean the difference between periods of bad asthma attacks and a normal life.

Q: What anti-inflammatories are available?

A: This class of medications includes **corticosteroids**, **cromolyn sodium** and **ketotifen**.

Q: What can you tell me about corticosteroids?

A: Many experts believe corticosteriods, commonly called steroids, are the most effective anti-inflammatory drugs in treating asthma. In fact, one 1992 study suggests that the use of inhaled corticosteriods reduces the risk of fatal or near-fatal asthma *tenfold*.

Inhaled corticosteroids come in several formulations: **beclomethasone** (Beconase, Beclovent, Vanenase, Vanceril), **flunisolide** (AeroBid, Nasalide) and **triamcinolone** (Azmacort, Nasacort).

Q: How quickly do inhaled steroids work?

A: Generally, inhaled steroids take one to four weeks to reach their full effect. After that, the lungs become less "twitchy."

Q: Aren't steroids dangerous?

A: Don't be confused by the word "steroid" as used in the tabloids and popular press. There are many types of steroids, and the corticosteroids used for asthma (technically known as glucocorticoids) are completely different from the anabolic steroids sometimes used by weight lifters and athletes interested in building muscle mass.

Inhaled corticosteroids are believed to be safe for treatment of asthma, as very little gets into the bloodstream to cause side effects. Research is under way to determine the long-term effects of high doses of inhaled steroids.

Corticosteroids also come in pill form and as injections, and those forms are more dangerous, which we'll discuss in a moment.

Q: Do inhaled corticosteriods have side effects?

A: Yes. They often cause a fungal infection of the mouth known as thrush. A simple preventive step is to rinse the mouth after each inhalation. Some people report an occasional cough or creaky voice after inhaling the aerosol.

Q: What about the effects of inhaled steroids on children?

A: This is controversial. Some studies associate inhaled corticosteroids with impaired growth and some mild suppression of the adrenal glands, which produce hormones. Other studies show that growth is merely delayed, not stunted.

Researchers are looking further into the effect of inhaled steroids on children. Until the answers are in, doctors and parents have to weigh the potential side effects against the severity of their children's asthma. Children with severe asthma may need inhaled steroids to prevent severe attacks and trips to the emergency room.

There's no doubt, though, that inhaled corticosteroids are safer for children (and adults) than steroid pills or injections.

Q: Tell me about oral steroids. When are they used?

A: When severe asthma flare-ups (perhaps brought on by illness) can't be controlled by inhaled steroids, a doctor may prescribe a "burst" of such drugs as **dexamethasone** (Decadron), **methylprednisone** (Medrol), **prednisone** (Deltasone), and triamcinolone (Aristocort). The goal is to halt severe inflammation, a job that oral steroids do with speed and ease, and thus prevent hospitalization. Once asthma is under control, the asthmatic person goes back to his regular maintenance therapy.

This use of oral steroids is called *short-term steroid therapy.* Usually, the person with asthma receives one dose of the oral corticosteroid each day for 3 to 10 days.

Q: Is there another type of therapy?

A: Yes. Oral steroids are also prescribed on a long-term basis for people with severe chronic asthma. Long-term therapy, as it's called, may require daily or alternate-day doses.

Long-term therapy is not undertaken without good cause. Oral corticosteroids taken over several months suppress the body's normal production of hormones. That suppression can last 3 to 18 months after the steroid is discontinued and might pose a problem during times of physical stress, such as injury or surgery. Hormone suppression can be minimized by taking oral steroids every other day instead of daily.

Q: How quickly do oral steroids work?

A: Very quickly. Relief comes in about 3 hours and peaks in 6 to 12 hours. For someone with severe asthma, they can be a godsend—albeit one with side effects.

Q: What are the side effects?

A: Short-term effects from oral steroids include increased appetite, fluid retention, weight gain, muscle weakness, acne, peptic ulcer, high blood pressure and moodiness.

In children, long-term use of oral steroids definitely stunts growth (in contrast to inhaled steroids, which appear to delay growth). In children and adults, oral steroids can lead to **cataracts** (a clouding of the lens of the eye that obstructs vision), ulcers, **osteoporosis** (loss of bone mass), high blood pressure and an impaired immune system. Prolonged daily use of oral corticosteroids is reserved for people with severe asthma (despite use of high doses of inhaled corticosteroids). And even then, the asthmatic person and her doctor should periodically attempt to reduce dependence on oral corticosteroids.

A word of warning: Never discontinue corticosteroids abruptly without a doctor's order. Generally, people must be gradually weaned off oral steroids. Suddenly halting their use could literally send the body into shock.

Q: Are there any anti-inflammatory drugs that do not contain steroids?

A: Yes. The most common is cromolyn sodium (Intal).

Q: How does cromolyn sodium work?

A: Scientists don't know exactly how cromolyn sodium works but they suspect that it "stabilizes" mast cells and prevents them from releasing inflammatory chemicals. Thus it is sometimes called a **mast-cell stabilizer**.

What scientists *do* know is that cromolyn is an important preventive drug. It's particularly effective in preventing airway narrowing triggered by exercise, cold air, sulfur dioxide and pollen when taken before exposure to these triggers. At the moment, it's the best medication for preventing exercise-induced asthma.

Q: How is cromolyn used?

A: Cromolyn must be inhaled at least 15 minutes before exercise or exposure to allergens. Once an asthma attack has begun, cromolyn is not effective as a bronchodilator. Some people with asthma take cromolyn up to four times a day as part of their asthma-maintenance program. It usually takes a month of regular use to determine whether cromolyn is effective; cromolyn doesn't work for every asthmatic person.

Cromolyn can be inhaled from a metered-dose inhaler, as a nebulized liquid or by means of a powder-filled capsule placed in a Spinhaler, a small device that punctures the capsule and propels the powder into the lungs. A new form of cromolyn, Gastrocom, is a powder that can be dissolved in water and taken as a drink.

Q: What are cromolyn's side effects?

A: They are very few. The most common is wheezing or coughing after inhalation of the powder, a problem that can be addressed by switching to a metered-dose inhaler. Throat irritation, dry mouth, nasal congestion and nose bleeding have occasionally been reported.

Because of its few side effects, cromolyn is often the anti-inflammatory of choice for children with allergies and mild asthma.

Q: Are any other anti-inflammatory drugs on the market?

A: A new drug called **nedocromil sodium** (Tilade) has preventive action similar to cromolyn and is used in the same situations.

Another newcomer is ketotifen, a nonsteroidal anti-inflammatory drug. Taken in pill form rather than being inhaled, this prescription drug is designed to reduce the frequency and intensity of asthma attacks. It also appears to act as an antihistamine. However, it does not treat attacks in progress or act as a bronchodilator, and it must be taken regularly for one to three months before it becomes fully effective.

Q: What are ketotifen's side effects?

A: Ten to 15 percent of adults using ketotifen and a smaller percentage of children experience drowsiness during the first two weeks of taking the drug. The drowsiness apparently wears off.

However, like any nonsteroidal anti-inflammatory, ketotifen may not be suitable for asthmatic people who have aspirin allergies or nasal polyps.

MUCOKINETIC DRUGS

Q: What are these?

A: Mucokinetic drugs help clear mucus from the lungs. One mucokinetic drug is **guaifenesin**, an **expectorant** (found in many cough and cold syrups) that enables an asthmatic person to cough up more mucus. Another mucokinetic is **iodinated glycerol** (Organidin). These two drugs occasionally cause nausea, vomiting or drowsiness.

Other mucokinetic agents include saltwater solutions that are sprayed into the nostrils; aromatic inhalants such as eucalyptus and menthol; hot, steamy liquids like chicken soup; and garlic.

ANTIHISTAMINES

Q: How are antihistamines used in asthma management?

A: Antihistamines are sometimes helpful for people with extrinsic, or allergic, asthma. Antihistamines relieve nasal congestion, sneezing and the **hives** that often accompany allergic reactions.

Antihistamines are a new avenue of research in asthma medicine, and scientists are looking at ways that this family of drugs can block severe bronchospasms.

Q: Whew! There are lots of forms of asthma medications. How do doctors decide which treatment path to recommend?

A: Until recently, asthma was seen primarily as the result of excessive bronchoconstriction in response to environmental triggers or exercise. It followed, then, that bronchodilators were the drug treatment of choice. However, in recent years scientists have learned that asthma is an inflammatory disease. And that realization led in 1991 to a radical shift in treating the disease.

Q: What happened in 1991?

A: That's when new asthma-management guidelines were issued by the Expert Panel of the National

Asthma Education Program, a committee representing 29 scientific, professional and consumer groups. Convened by the National Heart, Lung and Blood Institute, the National Asthma Education Program was designed to alert primary-care physicians to these major changes in asthma management.

Q: What do the guidelines say?

A: They stress the importance of controlling inflammation by means of anti-inflammatory drugs. In particular, the guidelines propose a "step-care" approach to asthma-treatment plans.

Q: Could you explain the steps?

A: Here's a summary:

Step one, for people with attacks of mild or intermittent asthma: inhaled beta-agonists used daily or as needed.

Step two, for people with moderate asthma who experience flare-ups more than twice a week: inhaled corticosteroids, cromolyn sodium or nedocromil used daily in addition to beta-agonists.

Step three, for people with severe asthma (asthma not controlled by the maximum doses of bronchodilators and inhaled corticosteroids or cromolyn): oral steroids in addition to inhaled corticosteroids or cromolyn and bronchodilators.

Naturally, the guidelines go into considerably more detail than we have space to cover here, and they suggest alternate drugs and dosing for both children and adults. But you get the picture: Doctors today are asked not just to treat the symptoms of asthma with bronchodilators; they must also address the underlying inflammation that puts the asthmatic person at risk of more frequent and severe attacks.

Q: Are doctors following these guidelines?

A: Experts assert that many doctors have not yet absorbed the message, meaning that asthmatic people are being undertreated with anti-inflammatory drugs like corticosteroids and cromolyn.

As evidence, these experts point to studies such as one in California that tracked physician prescribing habits based on hospital admissions and emergency-room visits for acute asthma. Only 19 percent of the asthmatic people—whose asthma was severe enough to take them to the hospital, mind you—were on corticosteroid therapy at the time of discharge.

Interviews with asthmatic adults admitted to the emergency room show that undertreatment is a particular problem in the inner city. One-third of the people interviewed were on anti-inflammatory drugs at doses too low to have an anti-inflammatory effect, and many people were overusing beta-agonists—up to 44 puffs in the day before emergency-room admission! "Over one-third of the patients contacted their doctors when they were having an attack, but the physicians were not aggressive enough when they prescribed treatment," noted Tina Harter, M.D., of Johns Hopkins University (*Medical Tribune*, June 10, 1993).

Q: Do all doctors agree with the guidelines?

A: For the most part, the guidelines are applauded by health-care practitioners. There are some critics: An article in the *New England Journal of Medicine* criticized the guidelines for defining disease severity primarily by the frequency of asthma attacks while "ignoring the far more dangerous elements of the intensity and duration of the [airway] obstruction" (December 31, 1992). Other critics would like to see the guidelines' recommendations put to the test via long-term clinical trials.

No doubt the guidelines will be refined in the future. But at the very least, the guidelines have sparked a debate about asthma care and have brought the disease to the attention of primary-care physicians.

Q: But what about the consumer?

A: From the consumer's point of view, the guidelines also offer important advice on self-care, which we discuss in Chapter 6.

5 IMMUNOTHERAPY

Q: What is **immunotherapy**?

A: Immunotherapy, or **desensitization therapy**, is a medical approach to treating allergies. It's based on the theory that if the body is gradually exposed to small doses of an allergen, the body may in time become desensitized to that allergen, so it will no longer trigger an allergic reaction.

Q: So why would **immunotherapy** be used for asthma?

A: For people with extrinsic, or allergic, asthma, there may be times when it is difficult or impossible to avoid triggers. If asthma medications cannot control asthma symptoms and if the cause of those symptoms is an allergy, then doctors may recommend immunotherapy.

Q: How do I know if I have an allergy that causes asthma?

A: As we saw in Chapter 3, doctors can perform several tests to detect the presence of allergies. Skin tests—

such as the scratch test, skin-prick test and intradermal test—are used to determine if your body has been sensitized to one or more allergens. A sophisticated blood test called the RAST (radioallergosorbent test) measures the amount (if any) of allergen-specific IgE antibodies in your blood.

Q: If I have allergies, then what does immunotherapy do?

A: When immunotherapy succeeds, it prevents the development of allergic inflammation and makes the bronchi less hyperresponsive. In short, it neutralizes the allergic response and turns off the inflammatory process.

Q: Will immunotherapy help everyone with extrinsic asthma?

A: No. Of the approximately 40 to 60 percent of asthmatic people with allergies, about half are appropriate candidates for immunotherapy.

Q: Why so few?

A: Immunotherapy must be used judiciously, the experts say. To be a candidate, the person with asthma must meet certain criteria.

Q: And those criteria are . . . ?

A: First, the person must have allergic asthma caused by one specific allergy. People who are sensitive to more than one allergen are less likely to benefit from immunotherapy.

At the moment, immunotherapy is most effective in treating asthma caused by pollen—particularly grass and ragweed pollen—dust mites, certain molds and cat dander. It is not effective with food allergies.

Q: And the second criterion is...?

A: Immunotherapy should be attempted only on people whose asthma is not sufficiently controlled by allergen avoidance and drug therapy.

That means that before someone gives immunotherapy a try, she first does her best to avoid the offending substance, and her doctor in turn carefully adjusts her asthma medications. These two steps can bring about enough improvement to make immunotherapy unnecessary, according to a 1993 study. In that study, 20 percent of patients with allergic asthma discontinued immunotherapy because their symptoms improved after their medications were adjusted.

Q: Are there any other criteria?

A: People should already have some control over their asthma. One way to determine this is through a forced expiratory volume in 1 second (FEV_1) test, which we discussed in Chapter 3. People with moderate to severe asthma whose FEV_1 readings fall below 70 percent of predicted values are *not* appropriate candidates for immunotherapy, according to the International Consensus Report on Diagnosis and Management of Asthma.

Q: Are there any age constraints in immunotherapy?

A: Provided they meet the criteria discussed above, children age five and older and adults up to age 50 can receive desensitization therapy.

Q: Exactly how does this therapy work?

A: Allergen extract is given in a series of injections, commonly referred to as **allergy shots**. The extract contains the specific protein that causes the allergic reaction.

Initially, each injection contains a very small amount of protein allergen. Over a period of months, larger amounts of the protein are gradually added to the extract until the person reaches the maximum dose, or "maintenance level," of allergen. Once the person has built up to the top dosage of allergen per injection vial, shots are administered less frequently.

Q: How frequently are injections given?

A: To start, maybe once a week. When the maintenance level is reached, injections are given every three or four weeks.

Q: Are shots given year-round?

A: That's the current trend. Nonasthmatic people with allergies may receive shots just during allergy season, perhaps three or four months a year. In asthma treatment, people receive shots year-round, so that an asthmatic response is avoided when the allergen is next encountered.

Q: How long are the shots continued?

A: Progress is evaluated after the person with asthma has reached maintenance levels—usually after six months or after two allergy-season cycles, depending upon the trigger. If asthma symptoms have not improved, then immunotherapy is discontinued.

If all goes well, however, the person with asthma then can continue monthly treatments for up to five years. And if he is lucky after those five years of injections, the relief achieved through immunotherapy will last for years after the shots are stopped.

Q: Are allergy shots safe?

A: For the most part.

Most reactions occur in the first 20 minutes after an injection, which is why you'll be asked to remain in the doctor's office after you receive a shot. Some people experience mild, **local reactions**—meaning the reactions occur around the site of the injection. Temporary swelling and redness are examples. An antihistamine or an aspirin usually relieves this minor discomfort.

Some reactions last more than a day or occur 4 to 12 hours after the injection. These delayed reactions may come in the form of headache, fever, lethargy or some wheezing.

Contact the doctor if you experience a lengthy or delayed reaction. It generally indicates that future increases in allergen dose must be made in smaller and more gradual increments.

Q: Some allergic reactions are severe, right?

A: Yes. The most severe reactions are not local but **systemic reactions**. Occurring immediately after an injection or several hours later, they can be life-threatening.

Q: What are the symptoms of systemic reactions?

A: They include chest tightness and a full-blown asthma attack, hives, stomach pains, difficulty in swallowing, fainting and nausea. An adrenaline injection, antihistamines and theophylline may be needed to stop a systemic reaction from progressing to **anaphylaxis**, or **anaphylactic shock**, a severe and sometimes fatal systemic reaction.

Although deaths from allergy shots are rare, most of these deaths "involved anaphylaxis and resulted from errors in labeling, lack of personnel skilled in handling the reaction or lack of resuscitation equipment" in the doctor's office, according to an article in *Medical Tribune* (July 22, 1993). For that reason, allergy shots should be administered only in a physician's office where facilities and trained personnel are available to treat any life-threatening reaction.

Q: If immunotherapy is a success, does it cure asthma?

A: No cure for asthma has yet been found. However, if allergy shots work well, they can reduce or eliminate the reaction to certain triggers as well as reduce the amount of medication needed to control the disease.

In one recent study of asthmatic people with ragweed allergies, two years of immunotherapy led to higher peak-flow readings and fewer emergency-room visits compared with other asthmatic people in the study who did not undergo allergy shots. The people on immunotherapy needed less than half the asthma medication of non-allergy-shot people, leading doctors to postulate that the cost of immunotherapy could be counterbalanced by lower medication costs.

Some physicians call immunotherapy an inexact and controversial science because they don't know in advance whether someone with asthma will benefit from a lengthy series of shots. But other doctors are enthusiastic about immunotherapy because when it does work, it can be an effective tool for treating extrinsic asthma.

6 SELF-CARE: PUTTING YOURSELF IN CONTROL

Q: From all that I've learned from this book, asthma is a complicated disease. Honestly now—will self-care really make a difference?

A: Absolutely. Unlike many other illnesses, *the control of asthma rests in the hands of the patient and her family.* Self-care is not just important, it's essential.

This chapter (and indeed, this entire book) is designed to help each person with asthma take charge of her own treatment. You should keep in mind that the overall goal is to control asthma so you can have a full, productive life.

Achieving this entails cultivating a partnership with your health-care practitioner, controlling or eliminating triggers, adopting an exercise routine, learning to manage stress and making a commitment to measuring your peak-flow rates. It also entails understanding the role of each of the medications you take and using (not overusing!) them in your overall strategy for good health.

Q: That's a lot of responsibility! Isn't there an easier way around all this?

A: Alas, no. The fact of the matter remains: Managing your asthma is demanding and, at times, difficult. For most asthmatic people, it's a daily, lifelong process.

But the alternative—neglecting the disease—can threaten your very ability to live and breathe on this earth. That's why most folks opt for self-care.

As we mentioned at the start of this book, the real goal is to control your asthma instead of letting it control you. And the encouraging news is that control is literally in your hands!

PEAK-FLOW MEASUREMENTS

Q: How is that?

A: We're referring to home peak-flow monitoring—that simple and objective means of measuring airway obstruction we've mentioned several times. With a portable peak flow meter, you can check your pulmonary function at home, in the office, on the road—any place and any time, as often as you wish.

Regular use of peak flow meters is particularly valuable for people with moderate or severe asthma, because the devices can detect a potentially dangerous situation known as progressive airway narrowing (that is, narrowing that develops very gradually) before the asthmatic person is aware of it. When noticed early, progressive airway narrowing can be countered by a change in medication.

Endorsed by the American Academy of Allergy and Immunology, which calls them "lifesaving devices," peak flow meters have recently become a mainstay of asthma-management plans.

Q: Who can use peak flow meters?

A: The American Academy of Allergy and Immunology says that children as young as five years old can use peak flow meters adequately. Researchers in London have used meters in children as young as three.

There's some dispute over the usefulness of routine peak-flow measurements in people with mild asthma. A study reported in the *British Medical Journal* (February 26, 1994) suggests that home peak-flow monitoring doesn't improve asthma management in many patients, but it does improve care in people whose disease is severe or difficult to manage. Peak-flow proponents respond by noting that regular self-monitoring certainly doesn't make asthma worse, and that it teaches anyone with asthma to be mindful of changes in breathing patterns so they can adjust treatment accordingly.

Q: How are meters used?

A: There's a knack to using peak flow meters, and it's best to get personal, hands-on training in their use. (Not all doctors and nurses know how to use these devices correctly—be sure your practitioner is experienced and qualified.)

Here's a summary of what you'll learn: Taking a deep breath while holding the meter in the front of the mouth, exhale hard, fast and quick. The marker on the meter's scale will give the peak flow reading. Set the marker back to zero, and repeat the process two more times. Record the highest reading in a notebook that serves as your asthma diary, or log.

Q: How do I use this information?

A: The National Asthma Education Program recommends comparing readings to a "traffic-light" zone system. Fine-tuned by your physician, the traffic-light system is built upon your baseline, or "personal best," reading. (In a minute we'll explain how personal-best measurements are made.) By comparing the present reading with the personal best, you and your physician get an indication of how well asthma is being controlled.

Q: What are these zones?

A: *Green* (which might indicate 80 to 100 percent of personal best) signals all clear. In general, this means that asthma is under control and the person with asthma can follow his maintenance medication plan. When green-zone readings are commonplace, the physician may suggest a reduction in medications.

Yellow (50 to 80 percent of personal best) signals caution. The yellow zone may indicate that you are in the midst of an asthma attack and that you need to take more medication. Continual readings in the yellow zone may indicate that, in general, asthma is not well controlled and drugs in the maintenance therapy may need to be increased.

Red (below 50 percent personal best) signals medical alert. A red reading calls for a quick-acting bronchodilator. If readings do not immediately rise and stay in the yellow or green zones, then a doctor must be notified.

Q: Are these colors already drawn on the meter?

A: No. You won't find these colors premarked on the peak flow meter, since what constitutes a green, yellow or red zone varies from person to person. You could, if you wish, mark your meter with colored tape or marker at the appropriate spots. Better yet, think of the traffic-light system as what it is—a metaphor designed to help you know when to take action.

Q: How often should I take a reading?

A: When using peak flow meters for the first time, people with asthma are often asked to take measurements three or four times a day for several weeks. Anytime they notice a change in breathing, they take a reading and record the number in their asthma diaries, also making notes about asthma triggers, symptoms, action taken, time of day, weather conditions, food eaten, exercise—any factors or situations that might affect asthma.

From this process come two things: first, information about asthma patterns (perhaps indicating nocturnal asthma, continuing asthma or exercise-induced asthma), and second, the person's personal-best peak-flow value. The personal best is the standard against which subsequent measurements are evaluated. It's usually the highest measurement achieved in the evening after a period of drug therapy.

Q: Must I always take measurements four times a day?

A: No. Once you have your asthma under control, your physician may suggest taking them twice a day—first thing in the morning and again 10 to 12 hours later. Measurements are usually taken before medication; some doctors request a second set of measurements after medicating to see if the drugs are doing the job they are supposed to do. The readings are entered in the asthma diary and compared with the person's personal-best values. As noted above, if the highest value is less than 80 percent of the personal best, then more aggressive drug therapy and daily monitoring may be indicated.

For people with well-controlled asthma, measurements might be taken only two times a week, preferably as morning and evening readings on the same day. People with intermittent or seasonal asthma may choose to measure peak flow only when they are exposed to triggers, such as allergens or infections. Your physician can give you guidance here.

Q: Peak-flow measurements sound simple enough. What do they achieve?

A: Since peak-flow levels often drop before a person notices asthma symptoms, the peak flow meter can predict asthma attacks. In that case, preventive medications can be taken or a doctor notified.

From monitoring peak-flow measurements at home and entering the results in a diary, a person with asthma becomes more knowledgeable about her condition and thus can actively participate in building a treatment plan. Daily measurements can help her doctor adjust medication as needed. Regular measurements detect early stages of airway obstruction and reveal day-night variations in lung function: Low peak-flow readings in the morning, called "early-morning dips," indicate airway hyperresponsiveness (a sign of inadequate control of asthma). Medications can be adjusted as needed.

Q: About my personal best—will that always stay the same?

A: Probably not. That's why the personal-best value is ideally reevaluated at least yearly—to account for growth in children and progression of disease in children and adults. Peak-flow measurements should also be correlated periodically with spirometry tests done in the doctor's office.

In short, peak-flow measurements provide objective criteria for planning, starting and even stopping treatment. The corresponding diary aids in unearthing and investigating specific allergens or irritants at school or work that worsen symptoms. Working in tandem, the peak-flow measurements and the asthma diary can help your doctor develop a better medication plan.

THE DOCTOR AND
THE MEDICATION PLAN

Q: I've been meaning to ask you—what type of doctor can best treat asthma?

A: Many people with asthma get excellent treatment from their primary-care physicians, who might be general practitioners, family-practice doctors, pediatricians or internists. Asthma is a fairly common disease, and many primary-care physicians have experience with it. Moreover, special reports—such as the National Asthma Education Program's *Guidelines for the Diagnosis and Management of Asthma* (1991)—are designed and published specifically to give primary-care physicians new insights into asthma management.

At the same time, scientific advances in understanding and treating asthma are occurring at a brisk pace, making it difficult for primary-care physicians to know everything about this field.

Q: Does that mean I must see a specialist?

A: It's likely that at some point you will visit a specialist. That might be a pulmonary specialist— a doctor who concentrates on respiratory and immunological problems—or an allergist—a doctor who specializes in allergy and immunology. In your travels through the medical system, you may also meet pulmonary nurse specialists, respiratory-care therapists and physical therapists, even nutritionists or dietitians—all of whom can help you manage your asthma.

Q: What should I look for in a physician?

A: As we see it, the ideal asthma doctor is one with whom you can freely discuss treatment and ask questions. It's someone who encourages you to be an active participant in your health care. In addition, the ideal physician knows that asthma is a fickle disorder that can fluctuate in severity, and understands that from one day to another your asthma symptoms can differ widely.

Avoid practitioners who insinuate that asthma problems are all in your head or who accuse you of malingering. Choose someone who views asthma as a challenge rather than a nuisance, as Maryann Stevens so aptly puts it in her book *Breathing Easy: A Parent's Guide to Dealing With Your Child's Asthma*. Stevens recommends that you ask the doctor how he intends to treat the disease. If he focuses on crisis management, you may have the wrong person, Stevens says. What you need is someone who views asthma management as a long-term partnership—someone who, at the start of each office visit, asks *you* questions to clarify your main concerns about and expectations for treatment.

Q: Is this what people mean when they speak of the doctor-consumer partnership?

A: Yes—doctor and consumer working for the same goals. In asthma treatment, it also means that the person with asthma, the person's family and the practitioner work together to develop an asthma-management plan.

Q: What is this management plan?

A: Ideally, it's a set of written guidelines that you carry home with you. Also known as a medication plan, these guidelines spell out how to detect and treat asthma attacks, when to seek emergency care, and how to recognize when everyday medications are inadequate.

Q: Can you tell me more about the management plan?

A: Certainly. It should be tailored to you, and it should be periodically revised and updated. Depending upon the type of asthma you have and its severity, the plan may include:

• A list of drugs that you take every day—your "maintenance therapy"—and a description of how and when they are used and what they are to achieve.

• A strategy for handling asthma attacks, including a specific definition of what is an asthma attack for you. That definition might be a peak-flow reading below a certain number, or specific symptoms that persist after you've taken certain medication. The strategy should spell out what additional medications to take, how to take them (orally, inhaled, nebulized or self-injected), when to call a doctor, what to do if the doctor can't be reached, and when to head immediately to an emergency room.

Q: Will the management plan tell me what to do when I'm ill?

A: It should discuss how to cope with illness, particularly with those viral infections that make asthma worse.

Also look for criteria for premedicating to prevent the onset of symptoms. People who experience exercise-induced asthma, for instance, need to take prophylactic (preventive) medications, such as cromolyn sodium, before they become active. Exposure to allergens, cold air or other irritants might also call for premedication.

Q: **What else might the plan include?**

A: It should address how long to stay on extra medication after illness or after an asthma attack. Even though you feel well, your lungs may still be twitchy, and so your doctor may advise staying on medication for several extra days.

The plan can also cover strategies for special events, such as where to get help when you are vacationing far from home. In short, the plan should include any information you need to help you control your asthma—after all, it's your plan. It should be customized to answer your questions.

TRIGGER AVOIDANCE AND CONTROL

Q: **Okay, I've mastered the peak flow meter, and I've got my management plan in hand. What's next?**

A: Avoiding or controlling exposure to allergens or irritants. Keeping your living environment healthy is a crucial step in controlling asthma!

Begin by keeping at least one room in your house scrupulously clean. Experts describe this as creating an asthma sanctuary. Usually, that room is the place where a person spends the most time—the bedroom. If you can make your whole house a sanctuary, that's even better.

Q: **How do I do create a sanctuary?**

A: The first step is to keep as many allergens and irritants out of the house and the bedroom as possible. During pollen and mold season, keep windows closed, especially in the bedroom. Seal central-heating and cooling-system ducts to keep allergens in other rooms from being blown into your sanctuary.

Tobacco smoke, smoke from wood-burning stoves and strong odors and sprays have no place in an asthmatic person's home. Don't use air fresheners, dust sprays or carpet fresheners, particularly in the bedroom. If you must use household cleaning sprays, insecticides or paints, then wear a high-quality dust mask or respirator. Better yet, have someone else do the spraying or painting.

Q: What about pets in the home?

A: Almost all asthma doctors advocate a pet-free home, although many physicians acknowledge that pets can relieve the stress that accompanies any medical condition like asthma. If the asthmatic person has a pet, specialists recommend that the pet be kept out of the bedroom and isolated to one or two rooms of the home, if possible. Another family member can frequently groom the pet out-of-doors and bathe it once a week. An asthmatic person should wash after handling an animal and avoid putting her face in its fur.

Q: What must I do to control dust mites?

A: Reduce the number of places where dust—and dust mites—collect. Here's how:

• Encase your mattress, box springs and pillows in airtight, dustproof covers (available from allergy supply companies) to keep dust mites from setting up shop in the bed. Seal the zippers with fabric-reinforced tape.

• Use synthetic instead of feather pillows. Foam pillows absorb sweat and thus encourage mite and mold growth, so encase them or replace them yearly.

• To kill mites in bedding, wash sheets in hot water (130 °F.) every week; wash blankets and mattress pads every two weeks. Washable floor rugs and curtains are better than heavy carpets and drapes. Carpeting laid on concrete is particularly bad because the dampness from the concrete encourages mite growth. If you have carpets, experts recommend that they be vacuumed daily. You can also purchase special carpet-cleaning solutions, called miticides, that kill mites or neutralize the allergy-producing substance in mite debris.

• Replace upholstered furniture with wooden, metal or plastic furniture. Laminate posters instead of using dust-collecting picture frames; remove stuffed animals, dried flowers, houseplants and knickknacks; and generally keep dust catchers to a minimum. (There's some evidence that mites on kids' toys—teddy bears and the like—can be killed by putting the toys in a freezer for several days.)

Q: Wow—that's a lot of work! Is it all necessary?

A: It is if mites, pollen, mold and other allergens found in household dust trigger your asthma. In addition, experts recommend damp dusting at least once a week and as often as once a day. Vacuuming should follow the same schedule.

Q: I've been told that I need a special type of vacuum. Why is that?

A: Most ordinary vacuum cleaners capture large dust particles but do not collect tiny aeroallergens, such as dander and pollen—the very things that people with asthma need to have removed. Instead, these cleaners kick fine dust particles into the air for up to an hour after vacuuming.

The exceptions are vacuum cleaners equipped with high-efficiency particulate air (HEPA) filters and central vacuum cleaners with dust collectors outside the home (such as in the garage). These are the best vacuums for asthmatic households.

However, if you don't have one of these fancy vacuums, there are other approaches. You can wear a good-quality dust mask while cleaning, or a nonasthmatic person can vacuum for you; an hour later, after the mobilized dust has settled, damp dust the room. Another approach is steam cleaning the carpets, which can reduce levels of mite allergen for up to six weeks. Unfortunately, steam cleaning doesn't remove or alter one of the toughest allergens to budge: cat dander.

Q: **How do I keep mold out of my home?**

A: The best approach is to keep humidity levels between 25 and 40 percent. Both mold and dust mites thrive when humidity goes above 50 percent.

In your quest to keep your home mold-free, pay close attention to humid areas: bathrooms, kitchens and basements. Use an exhaust fan or open window to remove bathroom humidity, and wash all tubs, tiles, toilets and shower curtains with mold-preventing solutions. In the kitchen, run the exhaust fan when cooking to remove water vapor. Empty trash containers frequently. And in the basement, use vinyl flooring instead of carpeting. Add a mold inhibitor to paint, especially when applied to concrete, stone, brick or cinderblock walls.

Q: **Would a dehumidifier help?**

A: Yes, as long as it is set for less than 40 percent humidity and is cleaned frequently. The coils and water collector in dehumidifiers can harbor mold if they are not properly cleansed.

Q: A friend has recommended that I get an air filter for my home. What will that do?

A: Air filters, or air-cleaning devices, can remove cigarette smoke, mold spores and animal dander as well as general household dust.

Three types of air-cleaning devices can aid in reducing aeroallergens. The first type, a mechanical cleaner, uses HEPA filters, which are replaced periodically.

The second type is an electrostatic precipitator, which places a static charge on metal plates. Dust particles passing through the machine accumulate on the plates via static electricity. The plates are cleaned frequently to remove the dust.

Both devices can be purchased as freestanding units or installed within heating and cooling systems. They can be expensive, and should supplement allergen control, not substitute for it.

Q: What's the third type of air cleaner?

A: Your basic room air-conditioner. It can do a great job of filtering air while at the same time reducing indoor humidity and making it more pleasant to keep windows and doors closed during months when pollen, mold and dust mites proliferate. Air-conditioners must also be cleaned periodically and their filters replaced.

Q: Let's say I've gotten my house in order. What can I do about triggers in the out-of-doors?

A: Admittedly, you can't control Mother Nature. When you're outdoors, you're exposed to ragweed, grass, pollens, molds and air pollutants. If these are especially troublesome, you'd be better off indoors, in an air-conditioned environment, particularly during the midday and afternoon, when pollen and some mold counts are highest.

You may be able to landscape around your house in a manner that discourages growth of irritant-causing plants. Avoid compost piles, mulches and piles of cut grass and fallen leaves. Have someone else mow the lawn. If you must mow it yourself, wear a pollen mask and shower promptly when the job is done to remove pollen and grass from your hair and skin.

EXERCISE

Q: Hold on here—I've got asthma. I can't exercise . . . can I?

A: Yes, you can. Asthma is no longer seen as a barrier to exercising. In fact, experts now urge all asthmatic people to incorporate daily exercise into their asthma-management plans.

Q: What does exercise do?

A: Exercise does many things, starting with an improved state of mind and greater muscle tone. Most of all for people with asthma, exercise builds lung strength and endurance.

Routine **aerobic exercise** conditions the body's muscles: It makes them more efficient at taking oxygen out of the blood. Eventually, the lungs don't have to work as hard to bring in additional air. In a person with asthma, this means that as his endurance increases, so does his maximum exercise capacity. He can exercise longer and more intensely, and exercise-induced asthma becomes less severe. This conditioning ultimately makes the lungs less sensitive to triggers.

Q: Aren't there certain sports that an asthmatic person must avoid?

A: No longer. Asthmatic people used to avoid strenuous activities, such as jogging, bicycling and cross-country skiing, because those activities require constant physical activity and thus are more likely to provoke bronchospasms. Today, with proper training and preventive medications, people with asthma can do intense aerobic exercise.

In fact, some researchers now say that asthmatic people wheeze and feel breathless when they exert themselves because they have been sedentary and are out of condition— not so much because of the severity of their disease. Certainly, asthmatic people do become breathless more quickly during exercise than people without the disease. But much of this can be combated by conditioning the body and using preventive medications.

Q: So how do I get started?

A: Check with your doctor before beginning a new exercise regimen. If you're out of shape, you might begin with a daily plan of exercise that requires short bursts of activity followed by a few moments of rest, such as doubles tennis, golf or bowling. Swimming has been described as the ideal sport for a person with asthma, because it is done in a warm, moist atmosphere. (Some asthmatic people, however, develop bronchospasms from the chlorine in pool water and thus must find another sport where they are not exposed to that chemical.)

Eventually you can enjoy walking, skiing, aerobics, baseball, tennis and squash—whatever you can handle, as long as it gets your heart pumping for 20 to 30 minutes and makes you work up a sweat. Such aerobic exercise builds cardiovascular fitness.

Q: What medications prevent exercise-induced asthma?

A: Cromolyn sodium, albuterol and metaproterenol are three asthma medications commonly prescribed for exercise-induced asthma. Generally, one of these is taken 15 to 30 minutes before exercise begins.

If you do feel your chest getting tight during exertion, you can try to work through these symptoms, or you can rest, take an inhaled bronchodilator and continue once the symptoms have disappeared (usually in 15 minutes). Exercise-induced asthma rarely appears again when the second period of exercise is within two hours of the first.

The premedication strategy applies to sexual activity also. Use a cromolyn or beta-agonist inhaler to improve breathing capacity and forestall asthma symptoms during lovemaking.

Q: Is there anything else I need to know about exercise and asthma?

A: Yes. If you plan a vigorous workout, do a 10- to 15-minute warm-up. After exercising, follow with a 10- to 30-minute cool-down of stretching or slow jogging. For cold-weather sports, wear a scarf or mask over your mouth to prewarm cold air.

DIET

Q: Are diets used in treating asthma?

A: Not really. Because asthma is a respiratory disease, food plays less of a role than it does in other disease—diabetes, for example. This is not to discount the importance of eating a nutritionally sound diet. Asthmatic people, like everyone else, need to keep their bodies healthy and fit.

That said, there are some instances where people have to adjust what they eat.

Q: Are you referring to people with food allergies?

A: Yes. Asthmatic people with food allergies or sensitivities may have to eliminate certain foods from their diets. As we mentioned in Chapter 2, tartrazine (yellow food dye #5) can induce asthmatic symptoms in some people, as can sulfites, which are food preservatives. Seafood, nuts and certain other foods have been linked with asthma flare-ups. For people with demonstrated food or medication sensitivities, reading food labels and asking questions at restaurants become survival skills.

Recently, several studies have linked a high-salt diet with asthma attacks in men. (Asthmatic women apparently don't experience any problems with salt.) Researchers suggest that it may be prudent for men with severe or unmanageable asthma to avoid high sodium intake.

Q: Can vitamin and mineral supplements improve asthma?

A: There is some research in this area, very little of it conclusive. Magnesium is a proven bronchodilator, and scientists are looking into its use as an adjunct to beta-agonists in treating moderate to severe asthma. Selenium appears to improve asthma, possibly by counteracting inflammation, but further studies are needed to make a clear connection.

Vitamin B_6 (also known as pyridoxine) was touted in the 1970s as a therapy for children with asthma. However, in 1993 it was clearly shown to have no benefits in asthma.

Q: I've heard about an herbal remedy from Japan that can control asthma. Do you know anything about it?

A: An herbal remedy known as *saiboku-to* is used in Japan to treat allergic diseases like asthma, according to a report in *Internal Medicine News & Cardiology News* (October 1, 1992). Known in the laboratory as TJ-96, *saiboku-to* is a form of *kampo*, traditional Japanese medicine based on herbal remedies. TJ-96 appears to exert the positive antiasthmatic effects of steroids but without steroids' side effects, and in Japan is used to control severe asthma.

"Traditional remedies of other cultures have often contributed significantly to modern medicine," the article notes. Scientific analyses of TJ-96 would be needed in the United States before it could ever be released for use here.

However, there's something very basic that anyone with asthma can drink to ease asthma symptoms.

Q: What is that?

A: Water. (We said it was basic!)
Dehydration sometimes occurs in asthmatic people, in part because the short, shallow breathing associated with asthma can dry out the lungs. Thus, people with asthma should sip water at the first sign of asthma symptoms and continue to sip it long after symptoms have passed.

Plenty of liquid can keep the body hydrated and thin mucous secretions so they can be coughed up more easily. Temperature can be important: Some people find that ice-cold liquids make asthma symptoms worse, and many children are bothered by hot drinks. For that reason, many doctors recommend that liquids be served lukewarm or at room temperature.

Q: What about drinking coffee or tea?

A: Coffee (and to a lesser degree, tea) is a beverage to consider drinking in an asthma attack. Although coffee is a diuretic, meaning it encourages the flushing of liquids from the body, coffee drinkers have one-third fewer asthma symptoms than noncoffee drinkers, according to the National Institutes of Health. That's because caffeine is a mild bronchodilator similar to theophylline.

Coffee is no substitute for asthma medication, and it can raise theophylline blood levels if you are taking that drug. But for many people with asthma, coffee can be used in a pinch if asthma strikes and your medications are not immediately at hand. Tea might serve the same purpose, though it generally has less caffeine than coffee. Check with your doctor to see if this tip would be useful to you.

PHYSICAL THERAPY

Q: I've heard that there are nondrug approaches to treating asthma. What are these?

A: The asthmatic person's chronically impaired breathing patterns may create other physical problems: a rigid, stiff posture that can result in rigid air passages and musculature; a weak diaphragm that results in less efficient breathing (specifically rapid, shallow breaths); and obstruction of air passages from excess mucus production. Physical therapy is sometimes used to combat these problems, and one of the most common physical-therapy techniques is called **postural drainage.**

Q: **What is postural drainage?**

A: It's a technique that uses gravity and **percussion—** gentle rapping on the chest—to loosen and eliminate thick, tenacious mucus. Generally performed by nurses and physical and respiratory therapists, postural drainage can be learned by family members and performed on an asthmatic person at home.

Q: **How is it done?**

A: The asthmatic person sits or lies in one of nine different positions, depending upon where mucus has collected in her lungs. The mucus is loosened by gently clapping, or "percussing," and then vibrating the chest with cupped hands. The goal is to enable the person with asthma to cough up mucus and mucus plugs that can lead to infection.

Postural drainage is performed only when a great deal of mucus is in the lungs. It is never done when the asthmatic person is in the midst of an asthma attack, because it could intensify breathing difficulties.

Q: **Are there other physical therapies to help people with asthma?**

A: Breathing exercises can increase muscle strength and even help relax the person with asthma. Some breathing exercises encourage slow, deep and controlled inhalations through the nose: Their purpose is to combat the asthmatic person's tendency to pant or breathe shallowly through the mouth, which can make asthma worse. Physical or respiratory therapists can demonstrate the appropriate technique.

Q: Must I always see a therapist to do breathing exercises?

A: No. You can do some breathing exercises without depending on visits to a physical therapist. Paul Sorvino, in his book *How to Become a Former Asthmatic,* describes twice-a-day breathing exercises that can be practiced in the home, including breathing games for children.

STRESS MANAGEMENT

Q: Is stress important to control?

A: Stress is not unique to people with asthma, but it plays a more complex role in the asthmatic person's life—it may trigger an asthma attack. So stress is something the person with asthma must reduce, if not avoid. This is easier said than done, as asthma itself—the whole impact of a chronic disease—can add stress to someone's life.

To help deal with tension and reduce the fear that an asthmatic person experiences during an attack, researchers are looking into techniques—variously termed "behavioral interventions" or "stress-management techniques"—as supplements to traditional asthma-management programs. These techniques can help the asthmatic person relax constricted muscles, combat stress and gain a sense of control over asthma as a disease.

Q: Can you give some examples?

A: Certainly. One relaxation technique used since the 1920s is called **progressive relaxation**. Others are **biofeedback**, **meditation** and **hypnosis**.

Q: What is progressive relaxation?

A: Also known as Jacobson's relaxation technique, it is based on the principle that someone can learn to recognize when particular muscle groups tense in response to stress.

Progressive relaxation is a sequence of gentle muscle exercises that alternately tense and relax the major muscles by groups. Progressive relaxation begins with the arms and hands, proceeds to the head and torso, and ends with the legs and feet. (Depending upon how it is taught, that sequence may be reversed.) Each muscle group is tensed for 5 to 10 seconds, then relaxed for 20 to 30 seconds. The idea is to observe the difference in sensation between tension and relaxation so that the person can learn to impose deep muscle relaxation in times of stress and anxiety.

Q: How does biofeedback control stress?

A: Biofeedback involves using sophisticated equipment and a technician who trains the patient to monitor, evaluate and alter a body process. In the case of asthma, biofeedback is used to facilitate relaxation training, lower pulse rate and control the opening of the airways, although there is no scientific evidence to show that biofeedback can really do the latter.

Actually another relaxation technique, biofeedback has made its way into mainstream medicine. Most major metropolitan centers have established biofeedback centers.

Q: You also mentioned meditation. How is that used in asthma?

A: Meditation combines breathing exercises and relaxation techniques. Research suggests that one form of meditation, transcendental meditation, lowers oxygen use, improves lung function and lowers heart rate.

Another form of meditation, **yoga**, combines gentle stretching and breathing exercises with the meditative state of mind. One small controlled study found that yoga can help people with mild asthma reduce their need for drugs and increase their exercise tolerance.

Q: And what about hypnosis?

A: Hypnosis is a trance state, similar to daydreaming, that combines heightened inner awareness with a diminished awareness of one's surroundings. Hypnosis can be used as a relaxation tool, teaching the asthmatic person to relax muscles and let go of anxiety. Some people learn to hypnotize themselves, and thus use self-hypnosis to relax and combat stress.

No one, however, can use hypnosis to make asthma go away. Hypnosis and other forms of stress management are adjuncts to—not substitutes for—medication and other self-care steps.

7 ASTHMA AND CHILDREN

Q: How common is childhood asthma?

A: Asthma is *the* most common childhood illness. In the United States, asthma and wheezing are among the top-10 reasons for visits to pediatricians, accounting for 2.2 million office visits a year. Five- to 17-year-olds in 1987 missed 10 million school days because of asthma and spent some 7 million days in bed.

Q: Is childhood asthma becoming more common?

A: Yes. During the 1970s, the prevalence of asthma in the United States increased 58 percent among 6- to 11-year-olds. From 1981 to 1988, asthma's prevalence in Americans under 18 increased another 40 percent.

Although the increase in the 1980s occurred exclusively among Caucasian children (for reasons unknown), asthma remains 26 percent higher in African-American children than Caucasian children and 12 percent higher in children who live in households with incomes below the poverty level.

131

Q: When does childhood asthma develop?

A: It can develop as early as infancy, although most childhood asthma appears between ages 2 and 5, which is when antibodies to inhalant allergens increase in a child's body. Childhood asthma is usually extrinsic, or allergic, asthma.

Q: Can a child outgrow asthma?

A: Some children who develop asthma in early childhood have fewer asthmatic episodes after age six, when smaller airways increase in size. About 50 percent of youngsters whose asthma began between ages two and eight experience an asthma-free period during their teens or early 20s; of those, half redevelop asthma in their 30s. As of yet, doctors have no way of determining which of these scenarios will apply to any particular child.

Regardless of whether a child outgrows asthma or must manage the disease throughout his life, the fact is that most asthmatic children lead full, productive and active lives. Asthma can be controlled, so that asthmatic episodes become a rarity and not an everyday event.

Q: Is asthma difficult to diagnose in children?

A: It can be. Before a doctor can make the diagnosis of asthma, she must rule out other conditions that have symptoms similar to asthma.

Q: Such as . . . ?

A: The so-called similar conditions include **croup**, an infectious disease common in children ages 3 months to 3 years; **epiglottitis**, an inflammation of the **epiglottis**, the cap that keeps food from entering the trachea; cystic fibrosis, a hereditary lung and pancreatic disease; and pneumonia, an inflammation of the lungs.

Bronchiolitis, an inflammation of the lining of the bronchioles common in infants, often heralds the onset of asthma and in fact is treated with asthma medications. Bronchitis may mimic asthma, and vice versa: **Cough-variant asthma**, in which the symptom is coughing rather than wheezing, can be mistaken for bronchitis. Even something as simple as a swallowed object can lodge in the throat or air passages and cause asthmalike symptoms.

The tests and procedures used to differentiate asthma from other conditions are discussed in Chapter 3.

Q: What are the signs and symptoms of childhood asthma?

A: Most are the same as for adults: wheezing, coughing, shortness of breath, chest tightness, rapid breathing and exercise intolerance.

In addition, an asthmatic child may have itchy, watery eyes; stuffy, runny nose; sore throat; dark circles under the eyes; flared nostrils; labored breathing; and hunched posture. Recurrent colds, flu, bronchitis or pneumonia may indicate asthma. Infants with asthma may refuse to suck, and may cough continuously, wheeze or generally act fussy.

Q: How is asthma in children different from asthma in adults?

A: The major difference is how fast asthma attacks can develop and worsen. Children have smaller airways that become obstructed much more quickly than those of adults. Breathing difficulties can quickly progress to medical emergencies. Thus, every asthma flare-up needs prompt attention.

Because attacks can happen quickly, it is especially important to control exposure to asthma triggers. Initially it may be a bit of a challenge to identify a child's triggers, particularly if the child is an infant. Keeping an asthma diary (see Chapter 6) can help with the detective work. Then, once the trigger is isolated, exposure to it can be reduced or eliminated.

Q: **Are certain triggers especially common?**

A: Triggers vary from child to child. They can include allergens, inhaled irritants, respiratory illness, exercise and the other triggers discussed in Chapter 2. However, one substance appears to increase the frequency and severity of asthma in most, if not all, asthmatic children.

Q: **And what is that?**

A: Cigarette smoke. According to one medical journal, asthmatic children who live in homes where parents smoke have three or four attacks a year that require medical attention. In contrast, asthmatic children living in smoke-free homes average only two such attacks.

"If parents of asthmatic children would stop smoking, it could cut the number of times their children have to seek medical help for asthma attacks by up to 80 percent," says James E. Haddow, M.D., of the Foundation for Blood Research, in Scarborough, Maine (*Medical Tribune*, July 8, 1993).

Q: Are there any special techniques for protecting a child from triggers?

A: You follow the same preventive strategies discussed in Chapter 6—removing triggers from the home (particularly the child's bedroom) and, whenever possible, restricting visits to places where triggers lurk.

Q: Should my child use a peak flow meter?

A: If your child is over age five, he or she may be ready to use a peak flow meter to detect changes in lung function that precede an asthma attack. Generally, children should use peak flow meters every morning and evening and whenever symptoms occur. Check with your doctor for recommendations on which type to purchase, and then follow the manufacturer's directions for proper use. Periodically check to see that your child is following directions properly.

The traffic-light zone system of interpreting peak-flow measurements, also discussed in Chapter 6, is very helpful for children.

Q: And again, that zone system says . . . ?

A: The green zone means all is well, yellow means caution (time to take medicine and watch for triggers) and red means red alert (call the doctor!).

Although you won't find these colors premarked on any peak flow meter (what constitutes a green, yellow or red zone varies from child to child), you could mark your youngster's meter with colored tape or marker at the appropriate spots. Better yet, teach your child to think of the traffic-light system as what it is—a metaphor to help her know when to take action.

Peak-flow measurements can help teach a child about cause and effect: The meter demonstrates how exposure to a trigger affects his ability to breathe fully and deeply, and so he learns why it is important to avoid triggers if he wishes to prevent the unpleasant experience of an asthma flare-up.

Parents like peak-flow measurements because these objective measures make it easier to determine when to administer medication and when to take their child to a physician.

Q: Are there other ways a child can participate in his own self-care?

A: Yes. At a very concrete level, he can take responsibility for filling in the asthma diary. In the doctor's office, he can participate in developing and adjusting the asthma management plan.

At a more abstract level, the child can learn how his disease works and learn to respect his limitations. In so doing, he becomes responsible for avoiding triggers, following the management plan, using medications as directed—in short, he learns to make informed and appropriate decisions about his health and his medical care.

Q: What if the child misjudges a situation and makes a mistake?

A: Mistakes happen. Triggers are not always controllable, and though most of the time kids won't do something that they know will make them feel lousy, willpower can waver. Next thing you know, the child with an animal-dander allergy has buried his face in a kitten, or the youngster with a grass-pollen sensitivity is knee-deep in a meadow looking for her baseball.

It happens. When it does, don't get angry and don't panic. Instead, turn to the child's asthma-management plan immediately.

Q: What can that do?

A: The plan might require giving the child additional medication and helping him relax until the medication takes effect, perhaps by giving him some soothing lukewarm liquids to sip. As we saw in Chapter 6, your child's plan will be customized to his or her needs.

Q: What happens if we follow the plan and an asthma attack still develops?

A: Call your doctor. Most physicians wish to be notified at the first sign of an attack—or anytime you have a health-care question, for that matter. Never feel shy about contacting the doctor's office! Although some asthma attacks are slow to develop in children, others progress rapidly.

In general, experts recommend that you call the doctor *immediately* if:

• Symptoms and/or peak-flow readings don't improve after the child has taken a bronchodilator.

• Peak-flow readings fall and do not respond to treatment.

• Peak-flow readings fall into the red zone—50 percent of personal best.

• The child has a high fever (over 101°F.).

• The child cannot walk, talk or play.

• The child is showing signs of obvious physical difficulty in breathing, such as hunched or lifted shoulders, or her rib cage and/or the neck around her Adam's apple is pulling in and out with each breath.

Above all, don't panic. Granted, that's an easy thing to say, but it is important to stay calm. Your panic might make the child fearful and anxious, and that extra stress could intensify an attack.

Q: When should an asthmatic child go to an emergency room?

A: Again, the child's management plan should spell this out, or the doctor should give you some instruction over the phone.

However, all experts agree that immediate emergency-room care is called for if the child's lips or fingernails have a bluish tint. This is a sign of a dangerous condition called cyanosis—insufficient oxygen in the blood. In such a case the child is experiencing a severe acute attack (*status asthmaticus* in medical lingo). Emergency-room or hospital care is needed to halt this attack, and we'll see in Chapter 8 how that is done.

Q: What medications can asthmatic children use?

A: Most medications for adult asthma are used for children, with adjustments in dosage and method of distribution. Generally, youngsters under age four or five can't use metered-dose inhalers (they can't coordinate medication release with inhaling it) unless a device called a holding chamber or spacer is attached to the inhaler. These devices slow down the medication jet and give a child more time to inhale the medication. Other options include using nebulizers (excellent for very young children) or taking medication in its syrup form.

Q: Which medications are commonly prescribed?

A: The answer depends on the type of asthma a child has (allergic, exercise-induced or another), the severity of the disease, the presence of other medical conditions, the child's age and other factors. Some youngsters find that certain medications are more effective for them than other medications. Some youngsters cannot tolerate particular drugs because, in them, those drugs produce bothersome side effects. Theophylline intolerances are common, for instance.

As you see, selecting medications is a rather complicated task, one that is part guesswork, part trial-and-error, part scientific knowledge. Fortunately, some guidelines give doctors a starting point for working out an individual child's medication plan.

Q: **What are those guidelines?**

A: Here are treatment recommendations, published in the *New England Journal of Medicine* (June 4, 1992), that are based in part on the National Asthma Education Program Expert Panel report.

Mild asthma (infrequent and brief symptoms): Infants and young children may be given inhaled beta-agonists as needed to relieve symptoms. If inhalers are impractical, then oral medications are used as needed. In children, inhaled beta-agonists may be given as needed.

Moderate asthma (symptoms more than twice a week): Infants and young children may be given cromolyn sodium along with theophylline or an oral beta-agonist. In children, cromolyn sodium, inhaled corticosteroids and theophylline may be given.

Severe asthma (daily symptoms): Infants and young children may be given inhaled corticosteroids and then, if needed, oral corticosteroids, in addition to medications listed above. In children, oral corticosteroids and long-acting oral beta-agonists (to control nocturnal asthma) may be given in addition to other drugs.

Q: **Does every doctor follow these recommendations?**

A: These are guidelines, not hard-and-fast treatment rules. An up-to-date physician will be familiar with them and take them into account when building an asthma-management plan.

Some experts suggest that these guidelines are a bit simplified. Whereas the three classifications—mild, moderate and severe—correlate well with the severity of asthma symptoms and medication requirements in adults, childhood asthma is harder to pigeonhole. Thus, treating children requires flexibility and awareness of situations that can change medication needs. Those needs can change as children grow older.

Q: You mentioned theophylline. I've been told that this drug creates learning and behavior problems at school. Is that true?

A: There certainly have been many reports that theophylline can make children hyperactive and less alert. But a recent study of 255 children is one of several that has laid some of that concern to rest. While the study did not dispute allegations that theophylline can change levels of alertness, it showed that such changes (if, indeed, they exist) had no impact on the results of scholastic-achievement tests.

In the words of the study's authors, "Academic achievement among children with asthma, at least those whose status is closely monitored in a structured treatment program, generally appears to be unaffected by asthma or by its treatment with appropriate doses of theophylline" (*New England Journal of Medicine*, September 24, 1993).

Q: And speaking of school, how can asthma best be managed in the classroom?

A: Pave the way for sound asthma control by giving teachers, school nurses and coaches a copy of the child's asthma-management plan. The plan should list your child's triggers; the symptoms of an asthma attack; what to do in response to symptoms or certain peak-flow readings;

your child's medications (including possible side effects); and who to contact in case of emergency. Above all, convey how important it is for teachers, nurses and coaches to respond quickly and calmly to an asthma episode.

Q: **Our school system requires that all medications be left with the school nurse. Is this common?**

A: Many schools set this requirement, which certainly makes it more cumbersome for a student to take her medication. Yet other schools allow students to carry and use their medications under carefully arranged circumstances.

If you think it is best for your child to have quick and easy access to asthma medications (particularly if she has had problems in the past), discuss this concern with school authorities. By law, schools are required to provide medical support for children with medical conditions such as asthma.

Q: **Which law is this?**

A: Ellie Goldberg, M.Ed., writing in *Understanding Asthma*, states that Section 504 of the federal Rehabilitation Act entitles all students with chronic illness—including asthma—access to necessary health services and gives asthmatic students the right to any necessary modifications in the regular education program. This means schools must work with asthmatic students and their parents to develop plans for those days when the children cannot exercise and plans for making up missed work caused by absences. Students should not be penalized for missing classes or gym because of asthma problems.

Official school policies or informal school practices that create barriers for students with chronic illness violate Section 504, Goldberg says. If there is a problem, talk with school officials. If the problem is not resolved, parents can dispute a school's action or refusal to act by contacting their state department of education or one of the U.S. Department of Education's Offices for Civil Rights.

Q: How do I know when I should send my child to school and when I should keep him home?

A: The International Center for Interdisciplinary Research on Immunologic Diseases at Georgetown University in Washington, D.C., has put together school-attendance guidelines for asthmatic children. These guidelines suggest sending a child to school if he has some nasal congestion but no wheezing, or mild wheezing that clears after he takes medication; if the child is able to do his usual activities; or if he has no difficulty in breathing.

On the other hand, the guidelines suggest keeping a child home if he has a viral or bacterial infection or a fever over 100 °F.; if he continues to wheeze an hour after taking medication; if he is wheezing too much or feels too tired to perform his usual activities; or if he has difficulty breathing.

Q: What about sports—how much can my child exercise?

A: For most youngsters with asthma, the sky's the limit. Doctors once advised selecting sports that do not require constant physical exertion but allow some respite (such as baseball, golf, volleyball, swimming). But as researchers, doctors and consumers alike learned about the role of warm-ups and premedication in averting exercise-induced asthma, those restrictions were lifted. Today's child is encouraged to pursue the sports she likes, as long as she realizes that participation in sports comes with certain commonsense caveats.

Q: Such as?

A: That she not exert herself in the midst of an asthma flare-up or when she is just recovering from a flare-up; that she stop exercising if she suddenly has trouble breathing; and that she exercise caution if peak-flow readings fall into the yellow zone or if she has been exposed to factors that trigger her asthma, such as allergens, air pollution, weather changes and colds or infections.

Q: Is there anything else a parent can do for a child with asthma?

A: Yes, and it's something many parents find difficult to achieve: Resist the temptation to coddle or over-protect an asthmatic child.

Q: What do you mean?

A: Here's what one mother has to say on the subject: In her book *Breathing Easy: A Parent's Guide to Dealing With Your Child's Asthma*, Maryann Stevens notes that the main obstruction confronting an asthmatic child is not a wheezing episode but the limitations imposed by concerned and fearful parents—restrictions that are frequently grounded in anticipated problems rather than real ones.

Although Stevens was talking about exercise, her words apply equally well to asthma management of children in general. Be careful in setting up a management plan that you build in restrictions based only on sound health care, not limitations based on fear. Unnecessary limitations make a child feel left out, even disabled. It can undermine his confidence in his ability to control his asthma.

To live full, productive and active lives, children with asthma need to participate in as many normal activities as possible, from chores around the house to fun-filled activities with friends.

8 WHEN TO SEEK EXTRA HELP

Q: Who needs extra help?

A: At one time or another, everyone with asthma needs special assistance in managing his asthma. That extra support might come in the form of an unscheduled trip to a doctor's office, a visit to an emergency room or a brief hospital stay.

Let's look first at the latter two scenarios: severe asthma episodes that require emergency-room care or hospitalization. Then we'll look at other situations in which the asthmatic person may need extra care: during surgery, pregnancy or advanced age.

ACUTE SEVERE ASTHMA

Q: What kind of asthma is this?

A: Acute severe asthma is a medical term for a sudden, serious attack that the person's usual medication is powerless to control.

It begins as a typical asthma attack with typical symptoms: wheezing, coughing, chest tightness and shortness of breath. These are all signals that the person's ability to breathe efficiently is impaired, something that a peak-flow measurement can confirm. At that point, he turns to his asthma-management plan. It may tell him to take additional bronchodilating medications (either by inhalation or via nebulizer) or to give himself an injection of epinephrine. Results should be seen quickly. Epinephrine, for example, usually breaks up a stubborn attack in three to four minutes.

Q: What if these steps don't work?

A: The initial asthmatic episode may worsen and progress to an acute severe attack.

The acute severe attack exhibits more dramatic symptoms: The person becomes anxious and apprehensive. Flaring nostrils and bulging neck muscles indicate that breathing has become hard work. The person sweats, his breath becomes shallow, his heart beats rapidly and his blood pressure may surge up and down. Initially he wheezes on exhalation, but as lung function deteriorates, wheezing diminishes and the person becomes speechless, physically exhausted and confused. The skin around his lips develops a purple tint, indicating insufficient oxygen in the blood.

Acute severe asthma is a medical emergency, and immediate emergency treatment is vital.

Q: Does an acute severe asthma attack develop quickly?

A: It may take a day, it may take hours or it may come on suddenly. Ideally, the person suffering the attack calls his physician as soon as he realizes that his backup medications aren't effective against the attack. The physician may direct him to a local hospital emergency department.

A handful of people with asthma experience attacks that progress from minimal symptoms to respiratory arrest— death—in one to two hours. This condition, termed **sudden asphyxic asthma**, illustrates how dangerous an untreated asthma attack can be. *Never hesitate to call your doctor.* If an attack progresses rapidly, head directly to an emergency room and call your doctor from there.

Q: How many people with asthma find themselves in emergency rooms?

A: About 12 percent of asthmatic people visit emergency rooms. Some experts believe that most of those people use emergency-room care repeatedly and fairly often.

Q: What happens in the emergency room?

A: If you go, you'll face a battery of tests and procedures aimed at assessing the severity of your asthma and stabilizing the attack.

Q: Would you describe these tests and procedures?

A: Here's a summary of what happens. The sequence of events and some of the procedures may vary, but you'll get the picture.

When you arrive at the emergency room (ER), you'll meet a triage nurse, someone whose job it is to judge the severity of an illness and allocate treatment. Tell the nurse how you feel. Summarize your medical history (mentioning any other medical conditions you have), explain what you have done to combat this attack (medication and self-care) and describe the ways in which this attack is more intense than usual.

An asthma attack merits immediate care. An ER physician should examine you very soon after your arrival. If not, be assertive, or have your advocate—a friend or family member —speak up. Make sure you get help right away.

Q: What will the doctor do?

A: The doctor's first goal is to evaluate the severity of the attack. She should review your medical history (the very same points you discussed with the triage nurse). She'll check your pulse and blood pressure, listen to your lungs with a stethoscope and ask you to do a pulmonary-function test. She may order chest x-rays and blood tests.

Q: Why blood tests when I'm having trouble breathing?

A: Blood tests help determine the cause of the attack and guide treatment. In particular, ER personnel need to know 1) how much theophylline is in your bloodstream, and 2) how much oxygen and carbon dioxide are in the arterial blood (that is, blood drawn from an artery in the wrist, not from a vein in the inner elbow). This second test, often referred to as the **arterial blood gas test**, is extremely important.

Q: What does an arterial blood gas test achieve?

A: It measures oxygen and carbon dioxide levels in the blood, which are indicators of just how severely the lungs are obstructed.

As you recall from Chapter 1, when airways are swollen or obstructed, air gets trapped inside the lungs behind the obstructions. The person having the attack breathes harder to force air through the blocked air passages. That may work for a while, but eventually the respiratory muscles tire from the immense effort. At that point, carbon-dioxide-laden air accumulates in the lungs, leaving less room for fresh, oxygenated air. As a result, the body cannot get enough oxygen or discharge enough carbon dioxide. The blood's oxygen levels plummet and carbon dioxide levels skyrocket.

Because this situation can be toxic, arterial blood gas measurements should be monitored throughout a severe asthma attack.

Q: Would I receive medication in the emergency room?

A: And then some. Even as the ER doctor is talking to you, ER personnel begin giving you asthma drugs. The first will be an injection of a fast-acting bronchodilator, usually epinephrine or terbutaline, to open up constricted air passages. Epinephrine, by the way, is not appropriate for people with high blood pressure, heart disease, a high pulse rate or a hyperactive thyroid gland. That's one reason why it's essential to give a brief medical history.

Next you may be asked to inhale a beta-agonist bronchodilator via a nebulizer, a machine that dispenses the drug as a medicated mist. When you're not using a nebulizer, you may be given oxygen (through a mask that slips over your nose and mouth or through a tube with prongs that fit into the nose) to increase the amount of oxygen that enters the air passages.

Finally, you'll be started on aminophylline, an intravenous form of theophylline. (This is why the ER staff needs to know how much and what type of theophylline you've taken in the past 24 hours.) Periodic blood tests monitor blood theophylline levels. Occasionally, someone with a severe cough is also given atropine (an anticholinergic bronchodilator) via nebulizer.

Q: Will these medications stop the severe attack?

A: Most of the time, but not always. If breathing has not improved in a half hour or less, ER personnel will administer epinephrine injections and nebulized beta-agonists several more times. These are in addition to the intravenous theophylline. You may be given an injection of a cortico-steroid if you are not responding to the other drugs.

Q: How long does all this testing and medication continue?

A: Within several hours it will be apparent if your asthma is stabilizing. When the ER doctor believes your lungs are free of obstructions and asthma symptoms are gone, she will send you home. Don't leave before you feel you are ready—your lungs are twitchy and vulnerable when recovering from a severe attack, and emergency treatment that is ended too soon can lead to a relapse.

Nor should you leave empty-handed. ER staff should give you specific instructions and perhaps medications (known as discharge drugs) for use in the next few days. They should also arrange follow-up care, either at a hospital clinic or with your physician. And, of course, you should discuss with your doctor everything about the attack and the way it was handled. The two of you may need to make adjustments to your asthma-management plan or improve some aspect of self-care.

Q: What happens if asthma doesn't stabilize in a few hours of ER care?

A: If your lungs haven't responded to the oxygen and asthma medications, you'll be admitted to the hospital. The admission diagnosis will be status asthmaticus: a severe, life-threatening asthma attack.

STATUS ASTHMATICUS

Q: How is status asthmaticus different from acute severe asthma?

A: There's a fine line between the two. Status asthmaticus is the more severe and dangerous form of asthma. The diagnosis of status asthmaticus implies that the person with asthma has not responded well enough to emergency-room care and that his deteriorated condition has become life-threatening.

Q: How is that?

A: Someone with status asthmaticus is on the verge of respiratory failure—meaning that his respiratory system is no longer able to bring in enough oxygen or discharge enough carbon dioxide from his body. This situation, as we've seen, can be toxic.

Q: What happens when someone is admitted to the hospital?

A: Care becomes more intensive. Staff members carefully monitor the person's respiratory functions, pulse and heart rhythm, and perform sputum analysis to unearth signs of bacterial infection. Additional blood tests detect the presence of eosinophils (specialized white blood cells that release chemicals causing inflammation in airway tissue).

Q: What medications are administered in the hospital?

A: In general, intravenous theophylline continues, with frequent blood tests to monitor blood theophylline levels; nebulized beta-agonists are given every few hours, as long as the beta-agonists don't dramatically increase the person's pulse; and large doses of intravenous steroids are given as often as every four to six hours. Antibiotics may be administered to clear up bacterial infections that develop around mucus plugs.

Q: Will people with status asthmaticus be given sedatives?

A: They shouldn't be. Sedatives and tranquilizers suppress the body's urge to breathe and to cough up mucus.

Q: What procedures are performed?

A: Procedures include a chest x-ray to locate areas of obstruction in the lungs and, in some cases, a procedure called **bronchial suctioning**, in which a thin tube is inserted into blocked air passages to remove mucus and mucus plugs.

The hospital staff continues to monitor arterial blood gases. Extremely low levels of oxygen and high carbon dioxide levels indicate respiratory failure, in which case the person is put on a machine called a **respirator**. Referred to as **mechanical ventilation** by the medical profession, the respirator's job is to take over the work of breathing. The respirator inflates the lungs at preset levels, giving the person's exhausted respiratory muscles a chance to recuperate while ensuring that his lungs receive enough oxygen. Mechanical ventilation may continue for several hours or several days.

Q: It certainly sounds like a lot goes on during hospitalization. Do complications ever occur?

A: They can. There's a small chance of injury to tissue along the air passages when hospital personnel insert or remove a respirator tube or bronchial-suctioning tube, or if the person coughs the tube out. Intubation may provoke bronchospasms in some asthmatic people. Other respirator-related problems include improper air temperature or humidity, and overventilation or underventilation of the lungs.

Other possible complications include pneumonia, low blood pressure and a collapsed lung.

Q: How many people are hospitalized with status asthmaticus?

A: About 500,000 people are hospitalized annually because of their disease, according to the National Institute of Allergy and Infectious Diseases. At least 10 percent of those admissions are for children.

Q: Which group is hospitalized more frequently— males or females?

A: That depends upon age. A recent study of 33,269 hospital admissions for status asthmaticus found that boys up to age 10 were admitted twice as often as girls the same age. Between ages 11 and 20, male and female admissions were nearly equal. Between 20 and 50, women were admitted three times more often than men; after 50, women were admitted 2.5 times more often than men (*Journal of the American Medical Association*, December 23-30, 1992).

Q: Earlier you described *how* an asthma attack turns into status asthmaticus, but what causes an asthma attack to worsen so dramatically?

A: Some doctors put the blame on the medical consumer: The person forgot to take his medication or ignored asthma symptoms or didn't call the doctor soon enough. But blaming the consumer is a simplistic—albeit, sometimes true—answer. Some of the blame lands on the shoulders of medical practitioners who do not take the time to develop written management plans for their patients, fail to give instruction in using devices such as inhalers and peak flow meters or do not keep up with the latest guidelines for asthma treatment (such as the regular use of anti-inflammatory medications).

Q: Can certain medical conditions cause attacks to progress to status asthmaticus?

A: There's mounting evidence that some people are physically unable to perceive asthma symptoms, particularly chest tightness, soon enough to prevent a severe attack. Many of these people have inherited an associated condition called **impaired hypoxic response**: Their bodies are less likely to notice a deficiency of oxygen reaching the tissues, and so their respiratory systems do not respond in ways to make up oxygen loss.

Together, reduced perception of chest tightness and impaired hypoxic response result in a delay in recognizing and treating an asthma attack. Experts believe these findings go a long way to explaining why 10 to 25 percent of asthma-related deaths occur within three hours after onset of an attack (*New England Journal of Medicine*, May 12, 1994).

These findings also illustrate why people with asthma should monitor their peak-flow rates regularly at home—particularly if they have had a history of emergency care—and should have a written management plan that spells out when to summon help. These folks should also wear a medical-alert bracelet and keep an epinephrine injection kit close at hand.

Q: Are some triggers more dangerous than others?

A: Yes. Some triggers—particularly adverse reactions to foods or drugs (see Chapter 2)—cause acute severe attacks, or sudden asphyxic asthma, in a matter of hours. Air pollution, even at levels deemed safe by federal air quality laws, can provoke serious asthma attacks, accounting for one in eight emergency-room visits for asthma.

Q: How can someone prevent a recurrence of status asthmaticus?

A: By promptly recognizing and treating any asthma symptoms in the future. As mentioned above, frequent peak-flow measurements and a revamped asthma-management/asthma-emergency plan are key. Careful avoidance or control of triggers and other preventive steps discussed in Chapter 6 lay a solid foundation.

Prevention is doubly important after the first instance of status asthmaticus. Statistics show that people who have been hospitalized with asthma attacks in the past have a higher risk of dying from asthma.

Q: Besides status asthmaticus, are there other risk factors?

A: There are several. In general, people who are at increased risk of asthma-related death fit one or more of the following descriptions, according to the National Asthma Education Program Expert Panel report and Francois and Sheila Sperber Haas in *The Essential Asthma Book*. Those at increased risk:

• Have had status asthmaticus in the past or have recently been treated for asthma in an emergency room or hospital.

• Have extremely low peak-flow readings each morning (what doctors refer to as "morning dipping," a sign of **labile**, or unstable, asthma).

- Have asthma that's been slowly getting worse.
- Take large steroid doses.
- Have asthma that began at a very early age, particularly before first birthday.
- Use beta-agonists excessively—well beyond recommended doses.
- Are noncompliant—refuse to follow a management plan or take medications as prescribed.

Q: Do other risk factors exist?

A: Yes. As we've mentioned elsewhere, issues of race, poverty and age also play a role. So do complacency and underestimation of the disease's severity on the part of the person with asthma, his family, his physician or his hospital. Significant depression, recent bereavement and unemployment and psychosocial problems, such as alcoholism and personality disorders, have also been linked to a higher death rate.

SURGERY AND ASTHMA

Q: Is there anything I should know about having surgery for medical conditions other than asthma?

A: People with asthma are at risk for certain kinds of complications during and after surgery, regardless of what the surgery is for. They include bronchoconstriction triggered by the insertion of a tube in the airways, **hypoxemia** (inadequate oxygen in the blood), **hypercapnia** (too much carbon dioxide in the blood) and atelectasis (collapsed area of the lungs).

It's common for people with asthma to have difficulty coughing up mucus after surgery, but coughing is important

to clear the lungs of mucus congestion. Thus, asthmatic
people are encouraged sit up, walk and otherwise move
around soon after surgery to break up congestion. In some
cases the doctor may recommend physical therapy, such as
postural drainage, a technique for loosening tenacious
mucus. (See Chapter 6.)

Q: I assume I should schedule elective surgery
when I'm healthy?

A: Correct. Schedule it well after a viral infection has
passed and not when you are experiencing asthma
problems. A checkup in your doctor's office can give you the
"all clear."

In the case of severe asthma, a physician may ask to admit
the asthmatic person a day or two before inpatient surgery
for a presurgical checkup, including such things as a chest
x-ray, pulmonary-function tests, arterial blood gas tests and
blood tests for infections.

Q: Are there complications related to
hospitalization itself?

A: Yes, infections.
Anyone who spends time in a hospital may acquire
a **nosocomial** infection—that is, an infection produced by
microorganisms that lurk within the hospital itself. People
with asthma are vulnerable to respiratory infections, which
can launch full-scale asthma flare-ups that last weeks or
months. A respiratory infection can be dangerous when the
person is recuperating from surgery.

The best precaution against the spread of infection is to
require that everyone—visitors, nurses, doctors, cleaning
persons—wash their hands before touching anything in the
asthmatic patient's hospital room, and that anyone with a
cold, flu or fever avoid the asthmatic person completely.

Q: How frequently do complications occur?

A: The likelihood of surgical or hospital-related complications depends on factors at the time of surgery: how sensitive the person's lungs are (*airway hyperresponsiveness*, as it's called), the degree of airflow obstruction and how much mucus is being secreted by the lungs. Obviously, a patient is better off if her breathing is stable and well-controlled as she goes into surgery.

Q: Is anesthesia a problem in asthma?

A: It is a concern. When possible and practical, the anesthesia of choice is local anesthesia, which numbs the surgical area and doesn't usually affect the asthmatic person's breathing. For many surgical procedures, including dental surgery, local anesthesia is effective and appropriate.

In contrast, general anesthesia causes loss of consciousness. An anesthesiologist controls the person's breathing by means of a breathing tube. There's always a small chance that the tube will irritate the airways, but general anesthesia poses less risk if asthma is stable before surgery.

Q: Will I need to take asthma medications while I'm in the hospital?

A: Yes, you must continue to follow your daily asthma-medication plan. The surgical team should maintain theophylline at proper levels throughout surgery. If you've been on corticosteroids in the past year, your asthma doctor may recommend a supplemental steroid "boost" before and after surgery.

Q: All this is fine for scheduled surgery, but what about emergency surgery?

A: You can increase the odds of getting appropriate medical care if you carry with you a wallet-sized medical-information card and wear a medical-information bracelet or necklace. These should state that you have asthma (and any other medical conditions), briefly list the medications you take, indicate whether you've been on steroids at any time in the past 12 months and provide your doctor's phone number or a number to call for details on your condition.

A medical-information card is a good idea for anyone with a potentially life-threatening disease.

Q: Are there other situations in which an asthmatic person needs extra care?

A: Yes. They include pregnancy and advanced age.

PREGNANCY AND ASTHMA

Q: What special steps are involved in treating asthma during pregnancy?

A: A woman with asthma who plans to become pregnant should first get her asthma under control, using the strategies we've discussed in this book, since her lungs must also provide oxygen for the unborn child. Well-managed asthma ensures an adequate supply of oxygen to the child and reduces the risk of complications during pregnancy, such as premature birth, difficult birth or an underweight infant. And the fact of the matter is, most women with asthma have uncomplicated pregnancies and deliver healthy babies.

Q: Does asthma worsen during pregnancy?

A: Approximately one-third of pregnant asthmatic women experience more asthma problems during pregnancy (usually women with moderate to severe asthma to start), one-third see no change in asthma symptoms and one-third find that asthma improves.

Asthma attacks in pregnancy should be handled with greater care: more frequent communication with doctors and greater attention to the asthma-management plan. Some physicians encourage more liberal use of office visits or emergency-room services so that asthma flare-ups can be treated more aggressively.

Q: Do medication needs change during pregnancy?

A: Medication use should be reviewed with the allergy doctor and the obstetrician or other birth attendant, as obstetricians prefer that pregnant women take the least amount of medication possible. Remember, though, that the key is to keep asthma under control, and medications are generally needed to avoid dangerous asthma flare-ups.

Q: Are asthma medications safe for pregnant women?

A: Most are considered safe, particularly in their inhaled forms, says the National Asthma Education Program Expert Panel report. Even corticosteroids can be taken, if absolutely necessary. Initially, theophylline doses may be lowered and then increased in late pregnancy to compensate for the mother's larger size.

However, certain medications are best avoided during pregnancy. These drugs are sometimes prescribed for people with asthma, although they are not asthma drugs per se.

Q: Such as?

A: Many cold and allergy medications are declared off limits because of some possibility of risk to the unborn child—an inconvenience for approximately 30 percent of women who develop hay fever during pregnancy. Hay fever is particularly bothersome for people with asthma, because it can bring on airway swelling.

Those off-limits cold and allergy medications include the antihistamines and decongestants brompheneramine and hydroxyzine (Vistaril, Atarax and Marax); alpha-adrenergic nasal decongestants (found in over-the-counter allergy or cold tablets); nasal sprays with epinephrine (Afrin, Neosynephrine, others); mucokinetic drugs with guaifenesin; and all medications containing iodine, such as iodinated glycerol, a mucokinetic.

Certain antibiotics should likewise be avoided, particularly ciprofloxacin, sulfur medications and tetracycline and its derivatives. But ampicillin, amoxicillin, cephalosporin, erythromycin and penicillin are safe during pregnancy, according to Stuart H. Young, M.D., in *The Asthma Handbook.*

Q: Is immunotherapy appropriate during pregnancy?

A: Many specialists believe that allergy shots can be continued without risk to the child if they were begun before pregnancy and if they improve control of the disease.

Allergy shots should not be started, however, nor should allergen doses be increased during pregnancy. There is no way to predict how a woman will react to a sudden increase of allergens in the bloodstream, and a severe, or systemic, reaction could cause a miscarriage or otherwise put the unborn child at risk. Likewise, immunotherapy that does not seem to make an improvement, or causes adverse reactions, should be discontinued.

Q: How is asthma treated after pregnancy?

A: The treatment often returns to that followed before the pregnancy. Women are encouraged to breast-feed their babies, as it's good for the health of the child. (Research suggests breast-feeding may reduce the chance that a child will develop allergies and/or asthma.) Mothers taking theophylline should watch for signs of irritability in the infant, an indication that dosage changes are in order.

AGING AND ASTHMA

Q: Okay, what about an area of concern further along the time line—asthma and aging?

A: Asthma tends to become more severe as a person ages. Statistics show that asthma-related deaths are highest among people 75 years of age and older.

Q: Why is that?

A: Researchers offer several reasons. For one thing, older asthmatic adults lose some of their ability to perceive one major asthma symptom: chest tightness. As a result, they are less likely to notice and treat breathing difficulties before attacks become entrenched.

In addition, older people, in general, lack the muscle tone and the cardiorespiratory reserve of younger people, and thus reach respiratory failure sooner.

Then there may be other medical conditions that make diagnosis and treatment of asthma difficult. Pneumonia, influenza and sinusitis, which are common ailments among the elderly, make asthma worse. Lifelong tobacco smoking can lead to emphysema in addition to asthma. And the longtime use of oral steroids to treat severe asthma can itself cause other health problems that affect asthma, such as gastrointestinal reflux and high blood pressure.

Q: Can't these other ailments be treated with drugs?

A: They can be and they are. But that opens another can of worms: adverse medication interactions.

Take high blood pressure, for example, which becomes more common after age 40. Estimates are that 35 percent of elderly Americans have high blood pressure. Some blood-pressure drugs, particularly a class called beta blockers, worsen asthma and shouldn't be used.

Other examples of interactions abound: Theophylline and epinephrine may aggravate heart conditions. Nonsteroidal anti-inflammatory agents used to treat arthritis can have a detrimental effect on an asthmatic person's breathing.

Q: What can an older adult do to guard against interactions?

A: Find a doctor who is sympathetic to the issue of asthma and aging and who keeps up with the latest developments in what is called geriatric medicine. Older asthmatic people react differently to treatments than younger people, and often need smaller doses of medication to achieve the desired response. The doctor you seek should be aware of new medications being developed to service more than one medical condition. For instance, two types of drugs, alpha-adrenergic blockers and calcium channel blockers, can improve both asthma and high blood pressure.

Q: Are there other special steps for the elderly?

A: Review the self-care strategies outlined in this book. An asthma diary can play an important role in detecting patterns and problems.

Also, make a special effort to guard against colds and flu. The elderly, in general, recover more slowly from respiratory infections, and for an asthmatic older person this is doubly true. Asthma-management plans need to offer several backup medications and strategies for keeping infections under tight rein. An annual flu vaccine and a pneumonia vaccination are wise preventive measures for older people with asthma— and for any asthmatic person prone to frequent respiratory infections.

Q: Acute severe asthma, pregnancy and asthma, aging and asthma—it all comes back to self-care, eh?

A: Yes. It's ultimately up to the individual to make the commitment to control his or her disease. By understanding the disease (especially the role of inflammation), controlling triggers, practicing sound self-care and forging partnerships with health-care practitioners, people with asthma can enjoy full, productive and active lives.

Q: What else can help me in this mission?

A: Keep asking questions—and get answers to them. Turn to the resources section of this book for a list of organizations that can guide you to more sources of information.

RESOURCES

Allergy and Asthma Network
Mothers of Asthmatics, Inc.
3554 Chain Bridge Rd., Suite 200
Fairfax, VA 22030
800-878-4403

American Academy of Allergy and Immunology
Allergy Information Referral Line
611 E. Wells St.
Milwaukee, WI 53202
800-822-2762

American College of Allergy and Immunology
85 W. Algonquin Rd., Suite 550
Arlington Heights, IL 60005
800-842-7777

American Lung Association National Headquarters
1740 Broadway
New York, NY 10019
800-586-4872

This number will refer you to a state chapter of this organization.

Asthma and Allergy Foundation of America
Information Clearinghouse
1125 15th St., N.W., Suite 502
Washington, DC 20005
800-727-8462

**National Asthma Education Program
   Information Center**
National Heart, Lung and Blood Institute
4733 Bethesda Ave., Suite 530
Bethesda, MD 20814
301-251-1222

**National Jewish Center for Immunology and
   Respiratory Disease**
Lung Line Information Service
1400 Jackson St.
Denver, CO 80206
800-222-5864
303-355-5864 (Denver area)

GLOSSARY

Acute severe asthma: Sudden, serious attack that usual medication is powerless to control; usually requires emergency treatment.

Adrenaline: See **Epinephrine**.

Aeroallergens: Allergens carried in the air, such as pollen, mold or dander.

Aerobic exercise: Steady activity that gets your heart pumping, conditions the body's muscles and makes you work up a sweat.

Albuterol: Beta-adrenergic agonist; used to open the airways.

Allergens: Substances that cause allergic reactions.

Allergic asthma: Another term for **extrinsic asthma**.

Allergic bronchopulmonary aspergillosis: Growth of mold spores in the air passages.

Allergic rhinitis: Hay fever.

Allergy shots: See **Immunotherapy**.

Alveoli: Tiny air sacs located at the tips of the bronchioles that play a key role in oxygen exchange.

Aminophylline: Xanthine drug; given intravenously in emergency rooms to open the airways.

Anaphylactic shock: See **Anaphylaxis.**

Anaphylaxis: Severe and life-threatening **systemic reaction**; also called anaphylactic shock.

Anticholinergics: Class of drugs that work as **bronchodilators;** also called parasympatholytics.

Antihistamine: Any of a number of compounds or drugs that counteract histamine in the body and that are used to treat allergic reactions and cold symptoms.

Anti-inflammatories (Anti-inflammatory drugs): In asthma, medications that prevent and reverse inflammation of the airways.

Arterial blood gas test: Measures oxygen and carbon-dioxide levels in arterial blood.

Asthma: Inflammatory disease in which air passages in the lungs periodically become narrowed, obstructed or blocked. Typical symptoms include shortness of breath, wheezing, chest tightness and coughing.

Atelectasis: Collapsed area of the lungs.

Atopic asthma: Another term for **extrinsic asthma.**

Atopic dermatitis: Long-lasting and sometimes severe skin condition.

Atropine: Anticholinergic drug; used to open the airways.

Beclomethasone: Inhaled **corticosteroid** drug; used to prevent or reduce airway inflammation.

Beta-adrenergic agonist: Type of **sympathomimetic** drug that opens the airways by stimulating beta-2 receptors in the lungs; also called beta-agonists, beta-adrenergic stimulants, beta-2 agonists or beta-2 sympathomimetic agents.

Beta-agonist: See **Beta-adrenergic agonist.**

Biofeedback: Stress-management technique that uses sophisticated equipment to train someone to monitor, evaluate and alter a body process, such as breathing.

Bitolterol: Beta-adrenergic agonist; used to open the airways.

Blind testing: Scientific challenge in which a person is given a dose of a suspected allergen or a placebo (a harmless substance) to determine if it triggers allergies or asthma.

Bronchi: Two air tubes that branch out from the trachea and in turn divide into smaller air passages.

Bronchial spasms: See **Bronchospasms**.

Bronchial suctioning: Procedure in which a thin tube is inserted into blocked air passages to remove mucus and mucus plugs.

Bronchial tree: Network of bronchi, bronchioles and alveoli that makes up the respiratory system.

Bronchioles: Smaller air passages that branch off from the bronchi.

Bronchiolitis: Inflammation of the lining of the bronchioles that obstructs the passage of air.

Bronchitis: Inflammation of the bronchi resulting in coughing and excessive mucus production.

Bronchoconstriction: Narrowing of the airways.

Bronchodilator: A drug that relaxes airway muscles, thus opening the airways.

Bronchoprovocation: Under medical supervision, deliberate exposure of a person with asthma to a suspected trigger to determine if the trigger causes airway obstruction and asthma symptoms; also called bronchial challenge or provocation test.

Bronchoscopy: Examination of the bronchi via a flexible fiber-optic tube (called an endoscope) that has been inserted down the throat.

Bronchospasms: Tiny muscle spasms or constrictions in the muscles that encircle the bronchial air passages resulting in airway narrowing.

Capillaries: Minute blood vessels that assist in oxygen exchange.

Cataracts: Clouding in the lens of the eye that obstructs vision.

Chronic asthma: Asthma that persists for a long period of time.

Chronic bronchitis: See **Bronchitis**.

Cilia: Delicate hairlike structures in the airways that filter air and clear out mucus.

Circadian rhythm: Body's natural 24-hour cycle, which causes fluctuations in the production of chemicals and hormones.

Corticosteroids: Drugs that prevent or reduce inflammation in the airways.

Cough-variant asthma: A form of asthma in which the symptom is coughing rather than wheezing; can be mistaken for **bronchitis**.

Cromolyn sodium: Inhaled **anti-inflammatory drug** that prevents inflammation in the airways; sometimes classified as a **mast-cell stabilizer**.

Croup: Infectious disease common in children ages three months to three years.

Cyanosis: Bluish-purple tint to the skin around the lips and under fingernails; indicates insufficient oxygen in the blood.

Cystic fibrosis: Hereditary lung and pancreatic disease that in children resembles asthma.

Dander: Pieces of sloughed-off skin from warm-blooded animals.

Delayed reaction or **response:** Asthma symptoms that occur 4 to 12 hours after exposure to a trigger; also called late response.

Desensitization therapy: A medical approach to treating allergies based on the theory that if the body is gradually exposed to small doses of an **allergen**, the body may in time become desensitized to that allergen so it will no longer trigger an allergic reaction.

Dexamethasone: Corticosteroid drug in oral form; used to reduce airway inflammation.

Dust mites: Microscopic creatures that feed on sloughed-off flakes of human skin; also called house-dust mites.

Dyspnea: Shortness of breath; difficulty breathing.

Electrocardiogram (EKG): Recording of the heart muscle's activity that is collected by electrodes placed on the chest.

Emphysema: Respiratory disorder in which the alveoli become permanently damaged.

Endoscope: Long, flexible fiber-optic viewing tube that enables a physician to look into a body cavity, photograph the interior and take a tissue sample.

Eosinophils: Specialized white blood cells that release chemicals causing inflammation in airway tissue.

Ephedrine: Sympathomimetic drug used less frequently today.

Epiglottis: Flap of skin that keeps food from entering the trachea.

Epiglottitis: Inflammation of the **epiglottis**.

Epinephrine: Sympathomimetic drug used in emergencies to open the airways; also called adrenaline.

Exercise challenge: Test to determine if exercise provokes asthma; type of **bronchoprovocation**.

Exercise-induced asthma: A form of asthma (with its accompanying symptoms—shortness of breath, chest pain or tightness, wheezing, coughing or endurance problems) experienced during exercise.

Expectorant: Mucokinetic drug or substance; used to loosen mucus from the lungs.

Extrinsic asthma: Type of asthma triggered by allergies.

Flunisolide: Inhaled **corticosteroid** drug; used to prevent or reduce airway inflammation.

Food challenge: Test to determine if certain foods provoke asthma.

Forced expiratory volume in 1 second (FEV$_1$): Test that measures the greatest amount of air that can be forcefully expelled in one second.

Forced vital capacity (FVC): Test that measures the total amount of air that can be exhaled as rapidly as possible.

Gastroesophageal reflux: Regurgitation of stomach acids into the esophagus; also called acid reflux or heartburn.

Guaifenesin: Mucokinetic drug and expectorant; enables the asthmatic person to cough up mucus.

Heart failure: Condition in which the heart's pumping ability has been impaired to a state of inefficiency that disturbs the entire circulatory system.

Histamine: Mediator released by mast cells during inflammation or allergic reactions.

Hives: Rash caused by an allergic reaction.

Homeopathy: Type of medicine that treats illnesses by using safe, natural medications that stimulate a person's own healing powers while avoiding harmful side effects.

Hypercapnia: Too much carbon dioxide in the blood.

Hyperresponsiveness: Airway narrowing that develops in response to exposure to allergens or irritants that do not affect the airways of nonasthmatic people.

Hypersensitivity: Overly sensitive reaction of the airways, sometimes referred to as lungs that are "twitchy."

Hypnosis: State resembling sleep that is induced by a person whose suggestions are readily accepted by the subject.

Hypoxemia: Inadequate oxygen in the blood.

Immediate reaction: Asthma symptoms that occur within 15 to 30 minutes of exposure to a trigger.

Immunoglobulin: Type of protein antibody released by the immune system to fight foreign viruses, bacteria, parasites or proteins.

Immunoglobulin E, or IgE: Type of protein antibody released by the immune system to fight against foreign viruses, bacteria, parasites or proteins; the major antibody in allergic reactions.

Immunotherapy: Antiallergy treatment in which a person with extrinsic, or allergic, asthma is given gradually stronger doses of allergen extract over a period of years. The idea is to desensitize the body to that allergen and thus prevent allergy-induced asthma attacks. Also called desensitization. Allergen-extract injections are called allergy shots.

Impaired hypoxic response: Condition in which the body is unable or less likely to notice a deficiency of oxygen reaching the tissues.

Intermittent asthma: Asthma with extended symptom-free periods and occasional flare-ups.

Intradermal test: Skin test in which an allergen-containing solution is injected directly into the skin.

Intrinsic asthma: Asthma that is not allergy related; also called nonallergic asthma.

Iodinated glycerol: Mucokinetic drug; helps clear mucus from the lungs.

Ipratropium bromide: Anticholinergic drug; used to open the airways.

Isoetharine: Beta-adrenergic agonist; infrequently prescribed.

Isoproterenol: Beta-adrenergic agonist; infrequently prescribed.

Ketotifen: Nonsteroidal **anti-inflammatory drug;** reduces the frequency and intensity of asthma attacks.

Labile: Unstable.

Larynx: Voice box.

Late response: Asthma symptoms that occur 4 to 12 hours after exposure to a trigger. Also called delayed response.

Local reactions: Generally mild reactions to allergy shots that occur around the site of the injection.

Lung volume measurements: Volume of air in the lungs during exhalation.

Mast-cell stabilizer: Drug that stabilizes mast cells and prevents them from releasing anti-inflammatory chemicals.

Mast cells: Type of cells found in the bronchial tree and elsewhere in the body; they release chemicals called **mediators** that provoke asthma attacks.

Maximum midexpiratory flow rate (MMEF): Test that measures how airflow decreases between 25 and 75 percent of the forced expiratory volume.

Mechanical ventilation: Process by which a respirator provides oxygen to a person's lungs.

Mediators: Chemicals that provoke airway inflammation, mucus production, bronchospasms and allergic reactions.

Meditation: Stress-management technique combining breathing exercises and relaxation techniques.

Metaproterenol: Beta-adrenergic agonist; used to open the airways.

Metered-dose inhaler: Device that houses a small aerosol canister filled with medication; dispenses precisely measured doses of medication as small puffs.

Methylprednisone: Corticosteroid drug in oral form; used to reduce airway inflammation.

Mold: Living organism that reproduces by producing microscopic spores that float through the air; also called mildew or fungus.

Mucokinetic drugs: Drugs that help clear mucus from the lungs.

Mucosa: Cells along bronchial airway walls. Also called mucous membrane.

Mucous membranes: See **Mucosa**.

Mucus plugs: Small chunks or spirals of mucus that collect in the airways.

Mucus stain: Analysis of mucus to detect the presence of **eosinophils**.

Nasal polyps: Grapelike protrusions in the lining of the nose.

Nebulizer: Machine that converts a solution into a fine, medicated mist that is slowly inhaled into the lungs.

Nedocromil sodium: Inhaled anti-inflammatory drug that prevents inflammation in the airways.

Nocturnal asthma: Asthma that worsens in the middle of the night.

Nonallergic asthma: Another term for **intrinsic asthma**.

Nosocomial: Refers to infections acquired during hospitalization, produced by microorganisms found in the hospital.

Occupational asthma: Asthma that develops from repeated exposure to one particular substance in the workplace.

Osteoporosis: Loss of calcium in bone mass, leading to weak and vulnerable bones.

Oxygen exchange: Process by which oxygen-rich blood gets to the heart and through the body.

Parasympatholytics: Class of drugs that work as **bronchodilators;** usually known as **anticholinergics**.

Peak expiratory flow rate (PEFR): Test that measures the maximum speed at which air leaves the lungs; also called peak flow.

Peak flow meter: Portable device used by people with asthma to keep track of their day-to-day peak-flow rates.

Percussion: Gentle rapping on the chest.

Pharynx: Throat.

Pirbuterol: Beta-adrenergic agonist; used to open the airways.

Pneumonia: Inflammation of the lungs caused by bacteria or viruses.

Postural drainage: Physical-therapy technique that uses gravity and gentle rapping on the chest to loosen and eliminate thick, tenacious mucus.

Prednisone: Corticosteroid drug in oral form; used to reduce airway inflammation.

Progressive relaxation: Sequence of gentle muscle exercises that alternately tense and relax the major muscles by groups; also called Jacobson's relaxation technique.

Prophylactic: Preventive.

Pulmonary embolism: Blood clot in the lungs.

Pulmonary-function tests: Tests that determine how well the lungs are performing and estimate the severity of airway obstruction.

Radioallergosorbent test (RAST): Test that measures the amount of allergen-specific IgE antibodies in the blood.

Respirator: Machine that takes over the work of breathing by providing oxygen and inflating the lungs at preset levels.

Respiratory failure: Life-threatening situation that develops when the respiratory system is no longer able to bring in enough oxygen to the body or discharge enough carbon dioxide from the body.

Reversibility: Symptoms that improve or disappear after medications are taken.

Reversibility test: Pulmonary-function test performed after the person with asthma takes asthma medication; determines if medication improves airflow.

Rhinoscopy: Examination of the interior of the nose and sinuses made by means a flexible fiber-optic viewing tube called an endoscope.

Salmeterol: Beta-adrenergic agonist; used to open the airways.

Scratch test: Skin test made with a series of short, superficial scratches on the skin, into which is rubbed an extract of a suspected allergen.

Seasonal asthma: A form of asthma that happens only at certain times of year.

Sinusitis: Inflammation of the mucous membrane of the sinuses, the open cavities behind the nose and eyes.

Skin prick test: Skin test in which a drop of allergen extract is placed on the arm and a needle pricks the skin under the drop.

Skin tests: Tests used to determine which substances, if any, cause allergies or sensitivities.

Spirometer: Computerized instrument that measures lung function.

Sputum: Material coughed up from lungs. Also called phlegm or mucus.

Sputum stain: Analysis of sputum to detect eosinophils, mucus plugs, destroyed airway cells, *aspergillus* mold and other information about the lungs' condition.

Status asthmaticus: Life-threatening asthma attack.

Sternum: Breastbone.

Sudden asphyxic asthma: Attack that progresses from minimal symptoms to respiratory arrest in one to two hours.

Sulfites: Chemical preservatives used to retard spoilage in certain foods, wine and drugs.

Sweat test: Test that analyzes salt content in sweat to diagnose cystic fibrosis.

Sympathomimetics: Class of drugs that work as **bronchodilators;** so named because they affect the sympathetic nervous system.

Systemic reactions: Severe reactions to an allergy shot or asthma trigger, such as **hives,** stomach pains, difficulty in swallowing, fainting, nausea and an asthma attack.

Terbutaline: Beta-adrenergic agonist; used to open the airways.

Theophylline: Xanthine drug; used to open the airways.

Trachea: Windpipe.

Triamcinolone: Inhaled **corticosteroid** drug; used to prevent or reduce airway inflammation.

Triggers: Substances or situations that provoke an asthma attack.

Ultrasound scan: Picture of organs and structures deep inside the body; made with high-frequency sound waves.

Ventilation measurements: Amount of air leaving the lungs and speed at which air is expelled.

Wheal: A temporary swollen lump in the skin, often accompanied by itching, tingling and burning.

Wheeze: Whistling or rasping sound heard during inhalation or exhalation; result of airway narrowing.

Xanthines: Class of drugs that work as **bronchodilators;** usually referred to as theophylline.

X-rays: Pictures of the body's internal structures made with electromagnetic rays with a short wavelength.

Yoga: Form of **meditation** that combines gentle stretching and breathing exercises.

SELECT BIBLIOGRAPHY

Altman, Lawrence K., M.D. "Rise in Asthma Deaths Is Tied to Ignorance of Many Physicians." *New York Times,* May 4, 1993: C3.

"Asthma Gene Find Met With Caution." *Medical Tribune* 33 (March 26, 1992): 33a.

Baker, Barbara. "Insidious Inhalers: Drugs for Asthma-Related Cough Can End Up Being One of the Causes." *Family Practice News* 23 (November 1, 1993): 3.

Barnes, Peter J., D.M., D.Sc. "A New Approach to the Treatment of Asthma." *New England Journal of Medicine* 321 (November 30, 1989): 1517-27.

Barnes, Peter J., D.M., D.Sc. "Blunted Perception and Death from Asthma." *New England Journal of Medicine* 330 (May 12, 1994): 1383-4.

Bone, Roger C., M.D. "A Word of Caution Regarding a New Long-Acting Bronchodilator." *Journal of the American Medical Association* 271 (May 11, 1994): 1447-8.

"Can Beta-Agonists Kill Asthmatics?" *Internal Medicine News & Cardiology News* 26 (August 1, 1993): 2,32.

Catterall, J.R., and Colin M. Shapiro. "Nocturnal Asthma." *British Medical Journal* 306 (May 1, 1993): 1189-92.

Clayman, Charles B., med. ed. *The Respiratory System.* Pleasantville, N.Y.: The Reader's Digest Association, 1992.

Faivelson, Saralie. "Patient Asthma Education Slows Revolving ER Door." *Medical Tribune* 34 (June 10, 1993): 2.

"Genetic Asthma Compound Found." *Medical Tribune* 34 (June 10, 1993): 11.

Gross, Kenneth B., Ph.D., et al. "Automobile Airbags May Cause Problems for Asthmatics." *American Family Physician* (September 15, 1993): 643.

Haas, Francois, and Sheila Sperber Haas. *The Essential Asthma Book.* New York: Charles Scribner's Sons, 1987.

Hogshead, Nancy. *Asthma and Exercise.* New York: Henry Holt, 1990.

Hurley, Dan. "Children of Smokers Have More Asthma Attacks." *Medical Tribune* 34 (July 8, 1993): 6.

Ince, Susan. "Asthmatics With Allergies Need Vigilant Shot Therapy." *Medical Tribune* 34 (July 22, 1993): 2.

Inlander, Charles B., and Paula Brisco. *The Consumer's Guide to Medical Lingo.* Allentown, Pa.: People's Medical Society, 1992.

Karr, Reynold M. "Occupational Asthma." *Immunology & Allergy Practice* 15 (February 1993): 17-20.

Knox, Alan J. "Salt and Asthma." *British Medical Journal* 307 (November 6, 1993): 1159-60.

Larsen, Gary L., M.D. "Asthma in Children." *New England Journal of Medicine* 326 (June 4, 1992): 1540-5.

"Life-Style, Not Asthma, Called Main Exercise Deterrent in Asthmatics." *Internal Medicine News & Cardiology News* 25 (July 1, 1992): 57.

Lindgren, Scott, Ph.D., et al. "Does Asthma or Treatment With Theophylline Limit Children's Academic Performance?" *New England Journal of Medicine* 327 (September 24, 1992): 926-30.

Lockie, Andrew. *The Family Guide to Homeopathy.* New York: Fireside/Simon & Schuster, 1989.

McCann, Jean. "Experts Say Asthmatics Still Being Undertreated." *Medical Tribune* 34 (May 13, 1993): 24.

McFadden, E.R., Jr., M.D., and Ileen A. Gilbert, M.D. "Asthma." *New England Journal of Medicine* 327 (December 31, 1992): 1928-37.

McFadden, E.R., Jr., M.D., and Ileen A. Gilbert, M.D. "Exercise-Induced Asthma." *New England Journal of Medicine* 330 (May 12, 1994): 1362-6.

McKeown, L.A. "Home Asthma Checks Urged." *Medical Tribune* 33 (September 9, 1992): 1,8.

Meier, Barry. "Company Tells of Dangers in Overusing Asthma Drugs." *New York Times,* August 8, 1991: A14.

National Asthma Education Program Expert Panel. *Executive Summary: Guidelines for the Diagnosis and Management of Asthma.* Bethesda, Md.: U.S. Department of Health and Human Services, 1991.

"New Asthma Regimen Increases Control." *Medical Tribune* 32 (April 4, 1991): 14.

Rudoff, Carol. *Asthma Resources Directory.* Menlo Park, Ca.: Allergy Publications, 1989.

Shayevitz, Myra B., M.D., and Berton R. Shayevitz, M.D. *Living Well With Chronic Asthma, Bronchitis, and Emphysema.* Yonkers, N.Y.: Consumer Reports Books, 1991.

Skobeloff, Emil M., M.D., et al. "The Influence of Age and Sex on Asthma Admissions." *Journal of the American Medical Association* 268 (December 23/30, 1992): 3437-40.

Sorvino, Paul. *How to Become a Former Asthmatic.* New York: William Morrow, 1985.

Spector, Sheldon L., M.D. "Asthma and Chronic Obstructive Lung Disease: A Pharmacologic Approach." *Disease-a-Month,* January 1991.

Spector, Sheldon L., M.D., and Nancy Sander, eds. *Understanding Asthma: A Blueprint for Breathing.* Arlington Heights, Ill.: American College of Allergy and Immunology, 1990.

Spitzer, Walter O., M.D., M.P.H., et al. "The Use of Beta-Agonists and the Risk of Death and Near Death From Asthma." *New England Journal of Medicine* 326 (February 20, 1992): 501-6.

Stephenson, Joan. "Immunotherapy Found to Benefit Asthmatics With Hay Fever." *Internal Medicine News & Cardiology News* 26 (May 1, 1993): 12.

Stephenson, Joan. "Used Judiciously, Immunotherapy Can Be Helpful in Allergic Asthma." *Family Practice News* 23 (May 15, 1993): 4.

Stevens, Maryann. *Breathing Easy: A Parent's Guide to Dealing With Your Child's Asthma.* New York: Prentice Hall Press, 1991.

"Subduing Nocturnal Asthma." *Internal Medicine News & Cardiology News* 25 (July 15, 1992): 1,41.

Weinstein, Allan M. *Asthma.* New York: Fawcett Crest, 1987.

Weiss, Kevin B., M.D., et al. "An Economic Evaluation of Asthma in the United States." *New England Journal of Medicine* 326 (March 26, 1992): 862-6.

Weitzman, Michael, M.D., et al. "Recent Trends in the Prevalence and Severity of Childhood Asthma." *Journal of the American Medical Association* 268 (November 18, 1992): 2673-7.

Young, Stuart H., with Susan A. Shulman and Martin D. Shulman. *The Asthma Handbook.* New York: Bantam, 1989.

Zoler, Mitchel L. "NIH Blitz Urges Altered Asthma R_x." *Medical World News* 32 (March 1991): 48.

INDEX

A

Absenteeism, asthma and, 22-23
Acetaminophen, versus aspirin and
  ibuprofen, 54
Acid reflux. *See* Gastroesophageal reflux
Acute severe asthma. *See also* Asthma attack
  death from, 147
  defined, 37, 145-46, 167
  emergency-room care and, 145-50
  signs/symptoms, 146
  status asthmaticus versus, 150-51
  treatment, 146-50, 164
Adrenaline
  defined, 81, 167, 170
  immunotherapy systemic reaction and, 106
Adults
  asthma in, 14
    versus children, 14, 133-34
    food allergies in, 52
Adverse food reactions, as trigger, 52-53, 124
Advil. *See* Ibuprofen
Aeroallergens
  air filters and, 120
  defined, 42, 167
Aerobic exercise, defined, 121, 167
AeroBid. *See* Flunisolide
Aerolate. *See* Theophylline
Age
  asthma and, 14, 27
  asthma and aging, 162-64
  immunotherapy and, 104
  intrinsic asthma and, 27
  peak flow meter and, 108-9
  respiratory failure and, 162
Air-conditioner, trigger avoidance and,
  116-17, 120
Air filter, types, 120
Air pollution. *See also* Smoke; Smoking,
  tobacco
  ozone and, 49
  as trigger, 23, 28, 48-49, 120
Airbags, asthma and, 48
Airflow obstruction
  bronchodilators and, 67-68
  x-rays and, 68
Airway hyperresponsiveness
  peak-flow measurement and, 112
  surgery and, 158
Airway inflammation. *See* Inflammation,
  airway
Airway narrowing. *See also*
  Bronchoconstriction
  mechanics of, 15-16
  peak flow meter and progressive, 108

Airway obstruction
  bronchoprovocation and, 72-73
  diagnosis of asthma and, 61-62
  exercise challenge and, 73
  peak-flow measurement and, 112
  tests for, 61-76
Albuterol
  defined, 81, 167
  versus ipratropium, 88
  nebulizer, 81-82
Allergens. *See also* Triggers
  asthma-management plan and, 115
  cockroaches, 46-47
  dander and saliva, 27, 29, 42, 44-45,
    117, 119-20
  defined, 27, 167
  dust mites, 27, 29, 42, 45-46, 57, 117-20
  generally, 27
  versus irritants, 46
  mold, 27, 42, 44, 116, 118-20
  pollen, 42-43, 116, 118, 120
  smoke, 49-50, 117
  tobacco smoke, 49-50, 117, 120, 134
Allergic asthma, defined, 26-27, 167
Allergic bronchopulmonary aspergillosis
  versus asthma, 62
  defined, 62, 167
  sputum stain and, 62
Allergic rhinitis. *See also* Hay fever
  defined, 57, 167
  as trigger, 57-58
Allergies
  atopic dermatitis and, 26
  children and, 27, 132
  food, 52-53, 124
  and predisposition to asthma, 25
  skin tests, 69-70, 101-2
  as trigger (*see also* Allergens), 23, 26-27,
    29, 42
Allergist, defined, 113
Allergy shots. *See also* Immunotherapy
  defined, 104, 167
  frequency/duration, 104-5
  reactions, 105-6
  safety, 105
Alpha-adrenergic blockers, 163
Alupent. *See* Metaproterenol
Alveoli, defined, 15, 167
Aminophylline
  defined, 84, 167
  emergency-room care, 149-50
Anaphylactic shock, defined, 106, 168
Anaphylaxis, defined, 106, 168
Anaprox. *See* Naproxen
Anesthesia, asthma and, 158